Human Factors
in Healthcare

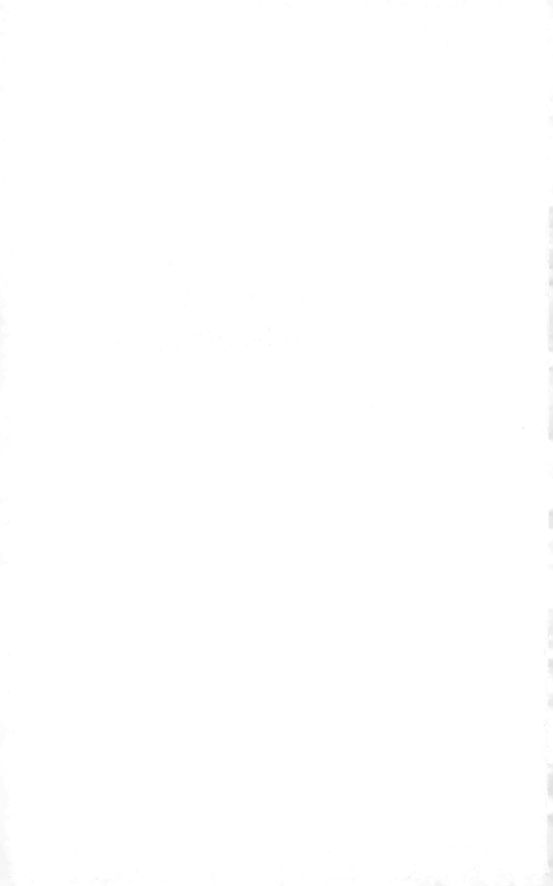

Human Factors in Healthcare: Level Two

DEBBIE ROSENORN-LANNG

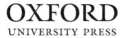

OXFORD
UNIVERSITY PRESS

OXFORD
UNIVERSITY PRESS

Great Clarendon Street, Oxford, OX2 6DP,
United Kingdom

Oxford University Press is a department of the University of Oxford.
It furthers the University's objective of excellence in research, scholarship,
and education by publishing worldwide. Oxford is a registered trade mark of
Oxford University Press in the UK and in certain other countries

Published in the United States of America by Oxford University Press
198 Madison Avenue, New York, NY 10016, United States of America

British Library Cataloguing in Publication Data
Data available

Library of Congress Control Number: 2015941611

ISBN 978-0-19-967061-1

Printed and bound by CPI Group (UK) Ltd, Croydon, CR0 4YY

Oxford University Press makes no representation, express or implied, that the
drug dosages in this book are correct. Readers must therefore always check
the product information and clinical procedures with the most up-to-date
published product information and data sheets provided by the manufacturers
and the most recent codes of conduct and safety regulations. The authors and
the publishers do not accept responsibility or legal liability for any errors in the
text or for the misuse or misapplication of material in this work. Except where
otherwise stated, drug dosages and recommendations are for the non-pregnant
adult who is not breast-feeding

Links to third party websites are provided by Oxford in good faith and
for information only. Oxford disclaims any responsibility for the materials
contained in any third party website referenced in this work.

To my sm

What have I learnt today and how can I share it?

Acknowledgements

Since I've finished writing this book, my patient and supportive childhood sweetheart has become my husband. I am eternally grateful for his encouragement and understanding. I am very lucky. Thank you, Steve, for being you.

Our six children continue to make me laugh and to teach me lessons daily about life. On the more challenging days, the motto that keeps me going is 'the harder the conflict the more glorious the triumph'. However, a single smile with a twinkling eye from one of them can melt away any dark moment.

I continue to value the support from my Mum, Sue, Jade, and Vaughan, and all of those mentioned at the beginning of the first book.

I would like to give a special thanks to Chris Gale for his help with the leadership chapter, and to Micky and Tanguy; their experiences and the learning I have drawn from it have been included.

I would like to thank Karen and Sara who listen and then nudge me along when needed!

Thank-you to all of those at NHS Education Scotland. I loved working with you and learned loads.

With thanks also to those at the Performance Coach for both the wonderful training you provided and for allowing me to include some of your materials within the book.

A final thank you to Caroline, James and Fiona from Oxford University Press for steering me through to the completion of this book. Thank you for your guidance and support.

Contents

1

Introduction

So many worlds, so much to do,
So little done, such things to be.
Alfred, Lord Tennyson, 1809–1892

Building on Level One

Can you remember something about a SHEEP? Do the terms G-NO-TECS, SBAR, SBIC, read back, cross check, and open culture ring any bells?

Level Two is designed to be read after the first book, Level One, as it will rely on that initial knowledge.

An understanding of the fallibility of human memory is often included in human factors training; I therefore start by highlighting some of the key principles from Level One by way of a refresher. I will, however, begin to introduce some new material at the same time.

Definitions of 'human factors'

We have established that there are many different enthusiastic scientific groups within the discipline of human factors in healthcare. For me, it is important that they are all embraced as they each bring a different angle to the solutions and the sum of the whole of all the solutions is far richer than taking any single slant. (I realize that I sound as if I am having a soap-box moment and I'm scarcely past the first paragraph!)

There are those who have a background in the pure science of human factors and ergonomics. There are those who started their working lives in the aviation industry and have now transferred their skills to healthcare. Some bring a background in psychology. Others, who work in multiple high-reliability sectors, are able to bring parallel experiences from different industries. Individuals with an informatics background will take a different approach again. Experience in simulation and education also plays its part. To my mind, all have a place and all should be welcomed.

It can be tricky to unite such varied expert views. Some view human factors as comprising non-technical skills, some as team training, and some as the

1

behavioural and attitude aspects of healthcare. Whilst I believe these elements are vital, this does not go far enough. There are many definitions of what human factors as a field actually is.

It is useful to remember the SHEEP model, which stands for *S*ystems, *H*uman interaction, *E*nvironment, *E*quipment, and *P*ersonal.

If you imagine knowledge and skills, 'human factors' are the ***glue*** that surrounds these and links them to:

◆ the *S*ystems within which we work,

◆ the people (including patients, their families, and staff) with whom we interact (*H*uman interaction),

◆ the *E*nvironment in which we work,

◆ the *E*quipment with which we work,

◆ and the *P*ersonal experiences and self-awareness that we bring to the workplace.

When we analyse errors we find it is this 'glue' that comes unstuck. A problem with human factors has been found to be responsible for around 80 per cent of errors in both healthcare and aviation alike.

Review of important concepts and models: SHEEP

In Level One we explored the sections of the SHEEP sheet in depth. The original SHEEP sheet has now been updated to SHEEP 2 (Figures 1.1 and A.1): Systems, Human interaction, Environment, Equipment, and Personal.

We started to try to shift the goalposts away from post-error analysis towards error prevention. This is tantamount to an alteration in philosophy to stop the proverbial horse leaving the stable rather than having to resort to a root cause analysis (RCA) to see how the horse got out and work out which door failed to close. I want to revisit the SHEEP model before we start to build on it.

Systems
Formal systems

In England, formal systems start with the Department of Health which sets targets and a general direction of travel. There are protocols and guidelines devised by various professional bodies about how we should behave (General Medical Council, Royal College of Nursing, etc.) and how we should treat specific conditions (various Royal Colleges and Associations, and national bodies). There are also central bodies that review the quality and standards that we are achieving (currently the Care Quality Commission and Monitor). There are educational and research bodies which have also been restructured recently. Each has its own guidelines and protocols and standard operating procedures (SOPs).

All these guidelines and protocols affect us and how we function but awareness of them and when they change is at best variable and at worst random.

Within some regional areas some of the organizations have power devolved to a more local level. There are some functions that sit with the organization itself and there will be an array of local systems guidelines, SOPs, and protocols too; some clinical, some human resources (HR), some IT, some financial, and so on.

Some of these local clinical guidelines replicate national guidance but add a local twist. Whilst I understand the need to make things relevant and encourage empowerment and ownership, I do not always understand the wisdom of this kind of reinvention of the wheel, especially one that has been designed by a panel of experts in the field. NHS staff often rotate through different organizations to gain experience. This means that they can be exposed to a variety of different versions of guidelines and policy. This at best causes challenges to adjust and at worst leads to ambiguity and error.

The challenge for each of us is to be aware of the systems and translate them so that they are relevant to us and to our teams. This involves being aware of when and where changes have been made and sharing relevant ones with the appropriate teams (for example, an issue with a medical device or a change in a resuscitation protocol).

Systems: The questions for you to ponder

Who is responsible for the information flow to raise the awareness of these changes at your departmental level and again at organizational level? When were your guidelines last reviewed? Are any out of date? Where are they stored? Can you access them in an emergency? What if the IT system was down, could you still access them now? How are new members of staff informed of them? How does a change get cascaded? How does your department share its learning after an error? How is this learning shared across the organization and beyond so that there is learning shared between organizations. What are your methods for improvement? How have your staff been empowered to produce local changes?

Do you have human factors education set up across your organization? Is it multi-professional? (In my opinion this is vital. We work together in a multi-professional arena and the learning of human factors is best achieved in those same multi-professional mixes.) I will devote the final chapter to my experiences and thoughts about how this is best achieved (Chapter 8). Do you have a

3

Systems

CULTURE

HOSPITAL CULTURE
- [ ] Departmental
- [ ] Professional
- [ ] Work group
- [ ] Mgmt vs. clinical
- [ ] Leadership culture

CULTURAL SYSTEMS LACK OF
- [ ] Open culture
- [ ] Safety culture
- [ ] Reporting culture
- [ ] Learning culture

INFORMATION FLOW
PROBLEM WITH
- [ ] Face to face
- [ ] Phone
- [ ] Written
  - [ ] Email
  - [ ] Text
  - [ ] Notes
  - [ ] Letter/fax
- [ ] Information gathering
- [ ] Access to info systems
- [ ] Access to info sets
- [ ] Briefing
- [ ] De-briefing
- [ ] Handover
- [ ] Info transfer between
  - [ ] Individuals
  - [ ] Departments
  - [ ] Organizations

INFORMATION SYSTEMS

MANUAL
- [ ] Patient notes
- [ ] Clinical pathway
- [ ] Care bundles

AUTOMATED APLICATION
- [ ] Theatre mgmt
- [ ] Bed mgmt
- [ ] Pathology
- [ ] Patient mgmt
- [ ] Radiology

INFRASTRUCTURE
- [ ] Network
- [ ] Hardware

PRESCRIBED (SOP/Protocol/Guildline Issue)
- [ ] Failure to follow
  - [ ] *National*
  - [ ] *Local*
  - [ ] *Legal & binding*
  - [ ] *WHO checklist*
  - [ ] *Care bundle*
  - [ ] *Research*
  - [ ] *Professional body*
- [ ] Lack of familiarity
- [ ] Different versions
- [ ] Ambiguity within
- [ ] Ambiguity between
- [ ] Unable to locate
- [ ] Chose to deviate due to
  - [ ] *Experience*
  - [ ] *Out of date*
  - [ ] *Inappropriate to situation*
- [ ] Refusal to use
- [ ] Complexity
- [ ] Not understood

MODELS/TOOLS
LACK OF USE OF:
- [ ] Productive ward
- [ ] TPOT (the productive operating theatre)
- [ ] Lean/6Sigma
- [ ] SBAR
- [ ] Read back
- [ ] Active identification
- [ ] Cross check
- [ ] Risk assessment
- [ ] Time checks
- [ ] Cognitive aids
- [ ] Site/side check

ORGANIZATIONAL FLOW
PROBLEM WITH
- [ ] Clinical Department
- [ ] Business Department
- [ ] HR Department
  - [ ] Recruitment
  - [ ] Retention
- [ ] Finance Department
- [ ] IT Department
- [ ] Discharge

Human interaction

TEAM DYNAMICS & CONFLICT

PROBLEMS WITH TEAM
- [ ] Personality types
- [ ] Unclear team roles
- [ ] Preferred team role
- [ ] Perceived unfairness
- [ ] Accountability
- [ ] Approach to change
- [ ] Difference in learning/communication styles
- [ ] Lack of support
- [ ] Mixed messages/ambiguity
- [ ] Assumptions

PROBLEM STAFFING THE TEAM
- [ ] Skill mix
- [ ] Staffing level
- [ ] Staff availability

CONFLICT
- [ ] Patient interaction
- [ ] Relative interaction
- [ ] Carer interaction
- [ ] Staff interaction

PROBLEM WITH
- [ ] Leadership styles
- [ ] Lack of leadership
- [ ] Lack of followership
- [ ] Hierarchy too steep
- [ ] Hierarchy too flat

LACK OF TEAM:
- [ ] Knowledge
- [ ] Skills
- [ ] Shared mental model
- [ ] Shared decision-making

BEHAVIOURS

INTERACTION QUALITY
- [ ] Failure to challenge negative behaviour
- [ ] Lack of diversity/prejudice
- [ ] Aggression
- [ ] Laziness/apathy
- [ ] Rudeness
- [ ] Snobbery
- [ ] Dishonesty
- [ ] Lack of consideration
- [ ] Lack of respect
- [ ] Over familiarity
- [ ] Empire building
- [ ] Trying to impress
- [ ] Negativity
- [ ] Unwillingness
- [ ] Fear/insecurity
- [ ] Malicious intent

TASK
PROBLEM WITH:
- [ ] Workload/multiple
- [ ] Tasks
- [ ] Prioritization
- [ ] Allocation of tasks
  Task:
  - [ ] Incomplete
  - [ ] Quality
  - [ ] Misunderstood

SITUATIONAL AWARENESS
- [ ] Loss of sense of time
- [ ] Failure to plan ahead
- [ ] Lack of care/compassion/dignity

PROBLEMS WITH COMMUNICATION QUALITY
PROBLEM WITH:
- [ ] Delivery of message
- [ ] Lack of clarification
- [ ] Duplication/ambiguity
- [ ] Listening ability
- [ ] Body language
- [ ] Language barrier
- [ ] Understanding
- [ ] Use of pronouns
- [ ] Memory
  Lack of:
  - [ ] Commentating
  - [ ] Option generation
  - [ ] Review of decision
  - [ ] Review of diagnosis

Environment

LOCATION CHANGE

PROBLEMS WITH JOURNEY BETWEEN LOCATIONS
- [ ] Complexity
- [ ] Distance
- [ ] Accessibility
  - [ ] Size
  - [ ] Secure areas
- [ ] Modality of transfer
  - [ ] Foot
  - [ ] Chair
  - [ ] Trolley/bed/stretcher
  - [ ] Vehicle
  - [ ] Lift/elevator
  - [ ] Lifting device (hoist)

INTERRUPTIONS
- [ ] People
- [ ] Bleeps/pager
- [ ] Phones
- [ ] Machines/equipment
- [ ] Media (text, email)

PHYSICAL
PROBLEMS WITH
- [ ] Atmospheric composition (air)
- [ ] Temperature
- [ ] Humidity
- [ ] Smell
- [ ] Lighting
- [ ] Noise
- [ ] Cleanliness
- [ ] Size
- [ ] Security
- [ ] Tidiness

ERGONOMICS

PHYSICAL DESIGN PROBLEMS WITH
- [ ] Infrastructure (walls etc)
- [ ] Immovable structures (cupboards)
- [ ] Movable structures (beds, chairs)

TASK RELATED DESIGN PROBLEMS WITH
- [ ] Resource location
- [ ] Knowing where it is
- [ ] Visibility
- [ ] Accessible
- [ ] Organised
- [ ] Standardised
- [ ] Optimised

SAFETY CONTROLS
- [ ] Radiation
- [ ] Electromagnetic field (eg MRI, laser)
- [ ] Biochemical hazard

FUNCTIONAL DESIGN PROBLEMS WITH
- [ ] Proximity to eating/resting/physiological function areas
- [ ] Privacy

VICINITY
- [ ] Arms reach area
- [ ] Immediate vicinity (no doors)
- [ ] Departmental area
- [ ] Hospital/GP practice/clinical unit
- [ ] External

Figure 1.1 SHEEP 2.

Equipment

GENERIC PROBLEM WITH EQUIPMENT ITSELF

- ☐ Fitness for task
- ☐ Manufacturing
- ☐ Supply
- ☐ Storage
- ☐ Availability
  - ☐ *Location*
  - ☐ *Not in stock*
  - ☐ *Timely access*
- ☐ Readiness for use
  - ☐ *Cleanliness*
  - ☐ *Working order*
  - ☐ *Maintained*
- ☐ Accuracy
- ☐ Reliability
- ☐ Safety
- ☐ Equipment compatibility
  - ☐ *Electrical*
- ☐ Safety coding
  - ☐ *Colour*
  - ☐ *Device interconnection*
- ☐ Model of equipment
- ☐ Equipment failure

CONSUMABLES

- ☐ Sterility
- ☐ Shelf life
- ☐ Administer
  - ☐ *Wrong patient*
  - ☐ *Wrong consumable*
  - ☐ *Incompatible*
  - ☐ *Left in patient*

DRUGS

- ☐ Prescribing abbreviated
- ☐ Prescribing illegible
- ☐ Prescribing wrong drug
- ☐ Prescribing wrong dose
- ☐ Prescribing wrong frequency
- ☐ Interactions between drugs
- ☐ Duplication
- ☐ Multiple charts
- ☐ Ambiguity
  - ☐ *Dispensing*
  - ☐ *Preparation*
  - ☐ *Administer*
- ☐ Wrong patient
- ☐ Wrong drug
- ☐ Wrong route
- ☐ Time delay
- ☐ Frequency
  - ☐ *Too frequent*
  - ☐ *Too infrequent*
- ☐ Wrong dose
- ☐ Wrong equipment
- ☐ Wrong technique
- ☐ Not available

NON CONSUMABLES

- ☐ Bed design
- ☐ Bed mechanical failure
- ☐ Bed electrical failure
- ☐ Bed mattress problem
- ☐ Bedrails
- ☐ Shower curtains
- ☐ Other

PROBLEM WITH USER INTERACTION WITH EQUIPMENT

- ☐ Knowledge/skill
  - ☐ *Training*
  - ☐ *Experience*
  - ☐ *Frequency of use*
  - ☐ *Familiarity*
  - ☐ *Ability to troubleshoot*
- ☐ Personal preference for equipment
- ☐ Availability of back-up equipment
- ☐ Ergonomic design/layout
  - ☐ *User interface*
  - ☐ *Ease of use*
  - ☐ *Complexity*
  - ☐ *Readability*
- ☐ Processing information
- ☐ Acting on information
- ☐ Post procedures check

INSTRUMENTS

- ☐ Sterility
- ☐ Administer
  - ☐ *Wrong patient*
  - ☐ *Wrong instrument*
  - ☐ *Incompatible*
  - ☐ *Left in patient*
  - ☐ *Wrong site/side*

MEDICAL GASES

- ☐ Prescribing
- ☐ Administer
  - ☐ *Wrong patient*
  - ☐ *Wrong gas*
  - ☐ *Wrong delivery method*
  - ☐ *Wrong time*

HUMAN TISSUE, BLOOD PRODUCTS & TRANSPLANTATION

- ☐ Collection
- ☐ Processing
- ☐ Prescribing
- ☐ Preparation
  - ☐ *Cross matching*
  - ☐ *Other preparation*
- ☐ Administer
  - ☐ *Wrong patient*
  - ☐ *Wrong blood/ product/organ*
  - ☐ *Wrong route*
  - ☐ *Wrong time*
    - ☐ *Point*
    - ☐ *Delay*
    - ☐ *Duration*
- ☐ Wrong dose

- ☐ Patient monitor failure

IMPLANTS/ PROSTHESES

PROBLEM WITH:
- ☐ Functionality
- ☐ Insertion method
- ☐ Wrong one
- ☐ Wrong site

2

Personal

EXTERNAL INFLUENCES

PROBLEMS WITH
- ☐ Mood
- ☐ Frustration
- ☐ Emotional security
- ☐ Emotional trigger (events)
- ☐ Feeling unprepared
- ☐ Failure to achieve expectations
- ☐ Lack of self awareness
- ☐ Confidence
- ☐ Self esteem
- ☐ Motivation
- ☐ Lack of interest
- ☐ Complacency
- ☐ Denial of the situation
- ☐ Adaptability
- ☐ Ability to cope with major change
- ☐ Distractions
- ☐ Coping with interruptions

PROBLEMS INFLUENCED BY WHO YOU ARE
- ☐ Race
- ☐ Gender
- ☐ Sexuality
- ☐ Age
- ☐ Personal value systems
- ☐ Personality (MBTI)
- ☐ Morals
- ☐ Cultural identity

PATHOLOGY/PHYSIOLOGY

- ☐ Tired
- ☐ Hungry
- ☐ Thirsty
- ☐ Toilet break
- ☐ Health/illness
  - ☐ *Physical*
  - ☐ *Mental*
- ☐ Stressed
- ☐ No energy
- ☐ Hormones/pregnancy

LIFE EVENTS

- ☐ Children
- ☐ Family
- ☐ Relationships
- ☐ Divorce
- ☐ Bereavement
- ☐ House move
- ☐ An argument
- ☐ Friends
- ☐ Commuting
- ☐ Parking
- ☐ Addiction to drugs
- ☐ Addiction to alcohol

ATTITUDES, BEHAVIOUR & EMOTION

MY WORK
PROBLEMS WITH
- ☐ An argument
- ☐ Poor morale
- ☐ Time pressure
- ☐ Lack of planning time
- ☐ Work time
- ☐ Rest time
- ☐ Work/rest balance
- ☐ Time of day
- ☐ Shift pattern
- ☐ Task conditions
  - ☐ *Elective*
  - ☐ *Scheduled*
  - ☐ *Urgent*
  - ☐ *Emergency*
  - ☐ *Clinical*
  - ☐ *Non clinical*
- ☐ High workload
- ☐ Lack of job satisfaction
- ☐ Job security
- ☐ Lack of team fit
- ☐ Lack of sense of belonging

human-factors champion? If not, will such a person come from patient-safety or quality improvement sectors? How will you integrate these three disciplines so that there is team working and not just repetition of functions or roles?

Informal systems

These include the culture within which we function. According to both Berwick and Francis, it is something we need to change. We will examine this more closely in Chapter 7.

Human interaction

It is quite common for people to use the term 'human-factors' training interchangeably with 'team training'. For me, team training is vital but it only one aspect (the H) of SHEEP, albeit in health arguably the most important.

What makes it particularly so in healthcare is the fact that the central part of healthcare is a person or a patient. This is different from areas where the field was originally studied—aviation and nuclear power—where an aeroplane or a nuclear reactor is the key component with which humans interact.

It is this vital human interaction between person and staff which needs improvement.

Both the Berwick and Francis reports have highlighted some improvements that are required. Human-factors training will underpin these improvements.

Each human interaction has complex components. For each individual within the interaction there are personality styles, preferred learning styles, preferred team roles, expectations, perceptions, values, past experiences, issues of culture, hierarchy, and more. All of these aspects are entwined within the interaction. We have highlighted the importance of self-awareness of your preferences in some of these aspects and how you may need to adjust your behaviour depending on with whom you are interacting. When you are working within your preferences, it will explain why you find it easier to work with some people rather than with others when you adjust your behaviours to fit in. It will probably explain who pushes your buttons and whose buttons you press.

Remembering that one can only alter oneself within an interaction and not the other person, I am sometimes asked 'why should I do all the ground work, shouldn't they meet me half way?' Wouldn't life be lovely if everything was fair! In an ideal world we would all work with insightful, self-aware people who are willing to adjust their personality preferences to work better with our own.

Those of us with at least some knowledge of these things may need to act as bridge builders. Why should we? For the benefit of the patients, staff, and the organization. Unresolved conflict or difficult interactions are distracting and make errors more likely. It is worth asking yourself, can you be the bridge builder?

Let us revisit the SHEEP sheet's H section (see Appendix 1, Figure A.1) as it is commonly some of these factors that go wrong. The largest source of error is communication, either between individuals or between professional groups or between clinical teams.

Briefing

We ought to begin every shift or episode of clinical care (briefing) by asking the question: where might today's error occur? This is sometimes referred to as 'where is today's gorilla or moon-walking bear'? (The relevance of these animals will be covered again in Chapter 2).

An example of a briefing that was widely introduced but only partially embraced is the World Health Organization's (WHO) surgical checklist. There are some organizations that have managed to persuade their staff of the importance of this briefing, bringing everyone on board with this culture change, whilst others have struggled. Some have variability; the checklist may be completed thoroughly in each step in some theatres but not in others, or it may be personality dependent (often influenced by the consultant surgeon responsible for the list). A checklist is only as good as the people that use it. If people engage fully with the checklist process it is very effective and has been shown to reduce error rates and improve patient safety, yet there are still mavericks out there who don't or won't follow the process. I cannot understand why; perhaps they think it is beneath them in some way? Some go through the motions but do so without being fully focused. I hope you will challenge this kind of poor behaviour if you come across it.

During the 'briefing' or 'huddle' or 'chat', or whilst 'boarding' (see definition in the next paragraph), it is worth reminding people about looking for potential risks that may lead to errors. If we notice the ticks on the SHEEP sheet starting to stack up, we can try to anticipate where the error may occur, hopefully in time to prevent it.

'Boarding' or doing a board round is simply a type of briefing performed by a large board, hopefully in a multi-professional group, where columns are provided for the patient's name, bed number, perhaps expected discharge date, and various tasks that might need to be performed. It offers an immediate visual representation of activities and whether they are completed. It should be clear to the whole team when processes are incomplete and help to prevent ambiguity and duplication. In some organizations, the interpretation of data protection rules has led to such boards no longer being placed where they can be viewed by patients and relatives. This can, however, have the effect of making them less accessible for the staff also and so some of the visual impact is lost.

Taking the moment to highlight the day's risks is often missed during these board rounds: a really valuable opportunity to be proactive in error prevention.

Example A 'The skill mix for this shift is not quite how I planned it as someone has gone off sick. Please make sure you come and find me if you have anything you aren't sure about.'

*Example B 'Please note there are two patients with the same surname today. Can we really make sure we are hot with our **active identification**.'*

Active identification

It sounds simple to make sure the correct patient is the one that is in front of you. Can you remember some of the factors that make the error of misidentification more likely?

Let's start with the personal ones from the P of SHEEP. If you are tired, under pressure (stressed or busy or high cognitive workload), under time pressure, distracted, interrupted—and for many of you that may just sound like an average day—you are at more risk of making a mistake.

The *S*ystem can also contribute to this error. By changing a list order or the order of a clinic or deviating from a routine way of doing things, this error can become more likely. So the next time you want to make some last-minute changes to the order of an operating list or a clinic or try to change a process in the interest of efficiency, stop. Take a moment to think and ask yourself whether your actions may precipitate an error.

By using this simple intervention, we can prevent an error occurring.

Step 1: Ask the person his or her name. This is not the same as you saying their name and asking them to confirm or deny it.

It should be: 'Can you please confirm your name?'

Not: 'Mrs Jones?'

Step 2: Ask the person his or her date of birth. Again he or she must say it, not you. But you should check it against your records as the patient tells you.

Step 3: Ask the person for his or her address. Check this against your records as the patient tells you.

Steps 2 and 3 may need to be modified to substitute hospital or NHS number, depending on what information you have available. I realize also that the patient may be unconscious or incapable of speaking, in which case check the name band against what is written in the notes.

These simple rules should be followed not only before a procedure but also for any consultation, be it in an outpatient clinic, a GP surgery, or a dental clinic. It may save the wrong patient being told that he or she has cancer, or the wrong tooth from being extracted.

Extra checks of identity should also happen prior to the administration of drugs and when prescribing, and to making sure blood results and X-rays belong to the correct patient.

Debriefing

We have explored the concept of a learning conversation at the end of every clinical episode or shift change or at the end of a non-clinical day (debriefing), where we can plant the seeds of an open culture. This conversation instils the thinking that 'continuous improvement' is normal for us, just an everyday occurrence. I might not call it a 'debrief'. I have found that it is more easily adopted if it is called something more informal, a 'chat', 'wash up', 'huddle', and 'take-aways' have all been adopted successfully.

I am sometimes asked questions about to how to apply this concept of a 'wash up' in other scenarios.

'I am a community midwife and I mostly work solo, how can I do a daily debrief?'

'I run a third of the hospital in my division, how can I do a daily debriefing of everyone?'

My answer is first that each of you is the expert in your own area of work. I hope that you will take these suggestions and adapt make them to your own circumstances, changing the bits that can be useful for you.

My thoughts on solo working are that of course this presents unique challenges. What about conducting a 'wash up' with yourself? Simply ask yourself at the end of every day 'what have I learnt today?' 'How can I share that learning with my peers and the wider team?' What about keeping a learning diary? Scribble a sentence in it at the end of every day that you think might be useful to share with others. When you meet up with your peers, be it daily or weekly or less frequently, take a few minutes to each share your top three learning points of the week.

Taking the other example, you personally cannot debrief an entire third of an organization. In this setting, there needs to be a cascade system along the lines shared in Level One. This is a debriefing system put in place at each local level and led by staff who are trained with the skills to extract lessons to be learned. Each leader for a local area meets, be it weekly or monthly, with his or her peer group and each member of the group shares a gem or two from their learning list. These are collected and passed further up the hierarchy to be shared there as well. But there should also be 'wash-up' sessions for the matrons and clinical leads and management layers. There should be continuing learning and improvement made at every level. Both the executive team and the board should also examine their own performance at the end of every meeting. The one question I would have them ask themselves is 'what value have we added to patient care today?'

We need learning to take place at every level, and a good question to ask is how might this take place across regions and throughout the country? How do executive teams and boards communicate what they have learned to competing teams and boards, I wonder?

We will explore a more detailed framework for a full learning conversation later (Chapter 5) where we will also discuss how to extract lessons safely after an error has occurred.

Different situations require different approaches to debriefing. Debriefing is not something you can just 'do'; like any other skill there is a learning curve and practice is required.

SBAR

In Level One we broke down the concept of information transfer into verbal and non-verbal components. We looked at the comparison of using verbal versus written information transfer, and at the hazards of using email, texts, written notes, or letters rather than speaking to someone face to face. We emphasized the importance of a structured handover tool such as SBAR: situation, background, assessment, and recommendation or request. We know that by standardizing the format for this information transfer we can improve the accuracy of the transfer. For more detail or a full refresher see Level One, Example 7.1, and the NHS Institute for Innovation and Improvement's Quality and Service Improvement Tools website for SBAR <http://www.institute.nhs.uk/quality_and_service_improvement_tools/quality_and_service_improvement_tools/sbar_-_situation_-_background_-_assessment_-_recommendation.html>.

SBIC

We introduced a tool for both delivering praise and challenging difficult behaviour, SBIC: situation, behaviour, impact, and change or continue (for more detail, see Level One, Chapter 3, pp. 72–5, section entitled 'Conflict resolution'; pp. 79–82, section entitled 'What to do when you are on the receiving end of poor behaviour'). A quick reminder of how to use the tool for either praise or challenge follows.

We have established that increased levels of praise can help to raise morale and that this, in turn, improves both morbidity and mortality.[1] However, praise should not be just a superficial 'thanks for doing a good job/working hard today', although this kind of comment is certainly better than nothing. Praise can be taken to a deeper, more meaningful level, where it will have more impact.

Situation: where are you going to have the conversation? Praising in public is useful (challenge should be conducted privately).

Behaviour: describe the behaviour that you witnessed (remember behaviour rather than the personality).

Impact: use an 'I' statement (e.g. I was proud/impressed/pleased/chuffed) and describe how you felt when you witnessed the positive behaviour.

Continue: encourage the person to repeat the same behaviour in the future.

Leading by example: Challenging poor behaviour

An aside:

When I refer to leaders in healthcare, I am thinking of a distributive leadership model with everyone leading their own part of the organization or process. The receptionist leading reception, the sister leading the ward, the porter leading his team, and the consultant leading hers. I am not simply referring to the Chief Executive and the executive team. Leaders who can generate a feeling that everyone, no matter what their job title or 'rank', takes responsibility for fulfilling his or her own role to the best of his or her ability.

As leaders, we are seen as role models. How we behave influences culture. If we are seen as failing to challenge poor behaviour we are seen as condoning it. Poor behaviour thus becomes part of the acceptable behavioural norms. We set the cultural barometer of the workplace. I have unfortunately seen many examples of very poor behaviour in healthcare over the last 20 years: bullying, shouting, throwing things, rudeness, and humiliation, or the more subtle behaviours of undermining someone, being work-shy, being a 'Mood Hoover', or ignoring someone. These behaviours often went unchallenged but now they must not.

Situation: choose a private place to have a conversation with the individual.

Behaviour: focus on describing the behaviour you have witnessed in a factual way without a judgemental tone. 'When you spoke to Mrs Brown's relatives … '.

Impact: use an 'I' statement, 'I was surprised, uncomfortable, troubled'.

Change: ask them, 'How else could you have handled the situation?'

Team training using the G-NO-TECS tool

In Level One we also explored a tool for generic non-technical skills (G-NO-TECS) (Figure 1.2), which provides us with a framework to introduce the concepts of team working, leadership, followership, decision making, task management, situational and self-awareness, and information management. It is a tool that has been developed for every member of the health service, no matter what his or her role. The tool can be used as a prompt for team training to introduce the concepts, or as a prompt for debriefing. It is not an assessment tool.

We will now build on these concepts and consider them in more depth in subsequent chapters dedicated to decision making, situational awareness, self-awareness, team working and 'followership', and leadership. A brief reminder is included here.

Situational awareness

When considering situational awareness, the triad of '*What? So what? What next?*' is a useful phrase to keep replaying to yourself. In other words:

What?

What are we dealing with here? What is the problem or working diagnosis?

So what?

S: Which guideline or process should we be using?

H: Who do we need for that? Are they here? Do we all know what we are doing (clear role allocation and competency for each role)?

E: Are we in the right place?

E: What equipment do we need? Is it all here?

P: Do I need any help? What are my stress levels like?

What next?

Will we need anything else, anyone else, or to move somewhere else? Is someone keeping track of time? Are we doing regular reviews to keep up with changes?

I teach DODAR in a slightly modified way from the original, but it is a good concise model to use.

Diagnosis

What is the problem? Even if it is as broad as 'this is an emergency', state it out loud to generate a shared mental model with those in the room.

Generic Non–Technical Skills (G–NO–TECS) Debrief Prompt[1]	COMMENTS

Team
 • Leadership skills (including approachability of leader)
 • 'Followership' skills (including assertiveness of followers)
 • Team building and maintaining (including hierarchy management)
     o Clear and appropriate role allocation
     o Consideration and support of others
 • Conflict solving	

Decision making • Problem definition and diagnosis (commentating, generating shared mental model) • Option generation (encouraging team input, avoiding fixation error) • Risk assessment and option selection • Regular review of decision as new information emerges	
Tasks • Providing and maintaining standards • Workload management (including distraction management and prioritization of tasks) • Knowledge of and ability to use equipment	
Awareness — Situational • Awareness of the systems • Awareness of the environment • Awareness of time (use of time checks) • Ability to plan ahead (anticipate need for staff/equipment/change of environment) • Maintenance of care, compassion and dignity **Awareness — Self** • Stress, fatigue, cognitive workload, time pressure, call for help if appropriate • Balcony and dance floor,[2] Swan	
Information Management • Gathering of information (from patient, relatives, team, other teams, records) • Sharing of information (including use of structured handover tool, e.g. SBAR) • Use of cognitive aids (guidelines, BNF, Internet) • Listening, non-verbal and verbal communication • Read back, active identification, cross check, open questions, avoidance of pronouns	

1. Source: data from Flin RH et al., Development of the NOTECHS (Non-Technical Skills) system for assessing pilots' CRM skills, *Journal of Human Performance in Extreme Environments*, Volume 3, pp. 95–117, Copyright © 2003.
2. Ronald A. Heiftze, Leadership without Easy Answers, Harvard University Press, Cambridge, MA, Copyright © 1994.

Figure 1.2 Generic non-technical skills (G-NO-TECS) debrief prompt.

Option generation

What else could this be? What possible management ideas should we be considering? Collect thoughts from the team.

'What else could it be?' and 'What am I missing here?' or 'Any other thoughts?' are useful questions to help people feel able to contribute their ideas.

Decide

Decide on a course of action and share this and the working diagnosis with the team.

Assessment

Continue to pull in more information from the history, examination, observations, and test results. Consider from where else you may be able to gather information.

Review

Continue to integrate the new information into the diagnosis and check whether it may need to be altered. Consider that the diagnosis is only ever the 'working' diagnosis, and continue to check that it is the correct one. Is the condition improving? Is the current management plan helping?

Return to D, diagnosis.

Revision of a few specific techniques

Read back

This is an easy technique to check that the transfer of information has taken place successfully between two individuals (see Example 1.1).

Example 1.1 Read back

Medical registrar (or equivalent grade as the titles seem to keep changing!):

'I need you to order an ECG on Mrs Wright, Mr Jones needs a chest X-ray, and we need to chase the thyroid function tests on Mrs Green.'

Foundation doctor replies: 'OK, that's an ECG on Mrs Wright, chest X-ray on Mr Jones, and chase TFTs on Mrs Green. Which ward was she transferred to?'

By repeating the information back, the sender gets to check that the information transfer has been successful and accurate. The receiver can also add any points for clarification (see Example 1.2).

Example 1.2 More read back

A: 'Please can you give 250 mls Hartmann's?'

B: 'Hartmann's?'

A: '250 mls now and then review vital signs.'

B: 'Giving 250 mls Hartmann's. How fast? And then repeat obs?'

Cross check

There is an important error that can occur as a result of expectation bias. This means you see what you are expecting to see rather than what is actually there. A technique that can help counteract this is a cross check. If I hold an ampoule of amoxicillin (an antibiotic) in my hand and I tell you that it is amiodarone (a drug used to treat abnormal heart rhythms), it is actually quite likely that you will read it as amiodarone. I am influencing what you are expecting to see; expectation bias. (Just *how* likely you will read it as amiodarone will be influenced by how busy we are, how well you know me and trust me, what has happened to you this morning, time pressures, and many more elements listed in the SHEEP-sheet boxes). On a more subtle level, what if I have picked up the right drug but of the wrong strength or concentration? If I hold a drug that has the right drug name but is the wrong strength and I confidently tell you that what I am holding is 2 per cent lignocaine rather than 1 per cent, it is even more likely that you will miss my error. My saying 'this is 2 per cent lignocaine' almost has an unsaid, 'isn't it?' tagged onto the end of my sentence. This can be referred to as confirmation bias, where I am asking you to agree with me.

The way to avoid this is the ***cross check***. When I ask you to check something, I simply ask you, 'what is this?' This open question does not alter your expectation of what you are about to see, but you have to engage in an active way to find out for yourself what it is that I am holding in my hand. In cross checking this way, we are much less likely to both make the same mistake.

The use of pronouns

There have been a number of terribly sad cases of mixing up two drugs where chemotherapy was involved. One of the drugs should be given into the spinal

15

fluid via a spinal needle and the other should be given via a cannula (a tube of plastic that sits in a vein) into the bloodstream. The wrong drug was administered to the wrong place, which had catastrophic consequences.

This particular error has subsequently been tackled in a number of ways. When considering error we use James Reason's concept using layers of Swiss cheese: only when the holes in the cheese line up can an error slip through our safety systems. A common approach following an error is therefore to put in more layers of safety (more slices of cheese).

In the chemotherapy example a systems approach has now been adopted so that there are more layers of safety in the process of administering these drugs. Rules have been introduced about the two drugs not leaving pharmacy together, about restrictions on who can administer the drugs and who can check them. There is an ergonomics approach being introduced where the end of the spinal needle will no longer fit a standard syringe and only drugs in a special syringe will be able to be attached to a spinal needle. The systems now in place are considerably safer than earlier versions, but however perfect you might feel your system has become, it is still possible for the layers of Swiss cheese to align on a bad day.

On one of those bad days a series of ticks lined up on the SHEEP sheet and despite all of those new systems being in place, the chemotherapy drugs both ended up in the same room with a person who had never given the drugs before and was being supervised by someone with more experience, but that person was on the end of a telephone.

We know that the chance of successful information transfer is reduced when using a telephone because there is no access to non-verbal communication (facial expression and body language is not available to add to the content of the communication). This applies to telephone conversations, e-mails, texts, and written notes.

The conversation that took place went along the lines of:

1. 'Has the drug arrived?'

2. 'Yes, it's here.'

3. 'Are you happy to give it?'

4. 'Yes, I'll give it now.'

'*It*', a simple pronoun, can be a dangerous word to use.

If the drug's name were to have been used, the ambiguity surrounding which drug was to be administered may have been removed and the error may not have occurred.

Opening up: Questions and suggestions

There are a number of questions or suggestions that can be used to help target specific items on the SHEEP sheet. It is often the person observing or someone not playing a central role in the process, and who perhaps does not feel responsible for the event that is unfolding, who sees the big picture. Alas, time and again we hear that the more junior members of the team, or those from a different profession, felt unable to challenge something they felt was going wrong (see the next section).

Here are some tips on ways to challenge that should feel safe to the challenger, no matter what role he or she is playing (see Table 1.1).

Table 1.1 Questions and suggestions

Tick on the SHEEP sheet	Question/suggestion to counteract it
No clear leader	'Who's leading?'
No clear team roles	'Who's doing what?'
Not using a guideline	'Which guideline are we using?'
No clear diagnosis or plan	'What's the diagnosis/plan?'
Self-aware but keen to avoid fixation error	'What am I missing here?' 'What else could this be?'
You think someone else might be fixated	'What's the working diagnosis? What else could it be?' 'What are we missing here?'
Leader appears out of his/her depth or is having a 'bunny in the headlights' moment	'Who shall I call for help?' or 'Let's get some more hands on deck. Who shall we call?'
Leader appears stuck or flustered	'Talk me through your thought processes', or 'Can we have a quick recap?', or 'What have we done so far?'
Communication breakdown—too quiet	'Talk me through your thought processes', or 'Can we have a quick recap of what each of us have achieved so far?', or 'What have we done so far?' 'Any thoughts on next steps?'

(continued)

Table 1.1 Questions and suggestions *(continued)*

Tick on the SHEEP sheet	Question/suggestion to counteract it
Communication breakdown—everyone is talking at once	'OK. I'm struggling to hear everyone, I'll come to each of you in turn. We will do this in a logical order starting with the airway, then breathing, then… So ….airway, give me an update.'
Inhibition of communication due to steep hierarchy	Leader needs to encourage ideas and contributions: 'What am I missing here?', or 'Any other thoughts?', or 'What haven't we tried yet?' Team need to be more assertive: 'Have we thought about…?' Or 'Could we consider…?' Or 'How about we…?' Or 'the guideline says we should …' (have the guideline in your hand)
Loss of sense of time	'How long have we been going now?' 'Who's keeping track of time?' 'Can you give me a time check every minute?'
Trying to put forward an idea but not being heard	Try to establish eye contact. Call the person by name. 'The tracheostomy set is ready.' Repeat, consider more volume. 'The tracheostomy set is ready, I am opening it now.' 'Can you repeat that back to me so that I know you have heard me?'

Hierarchy

Healthcare has a long history and it is heavily steeped in tradition and a well-established hierarchy. There is a structural hierarchy but, in addition, there is a difference in perceived power. This sense of perceived steep power differential seems well ingrained within some clinical areas more than others. This can be felt within a professional group (e.g. medical student to consultant or e.g.2 student nurse to sister-in-charge) or between professional groups, when an 'us and them' attitude is easily adopted.

This might refer to doctors and nurses, clinical and non-clinical staff (referred to as 'the management', or perhaps 'the Trust', or just 'them',' or even 'the dark side'), or primary and secondary care staff, or commissioners and providers, and so on. I find the multi-professional approach to education a good forum for asking, 'who are *they*?' and to try to move towards thinking in terms of 'we'. It is the 'we' who are trying to do the best for people/patients. 'We' are on the same side. I profoundly believe that only when we start educating people in this kind of forum and naming some of these kinds of issues can we start to remove some of the barriers.

Anecdote

There was a picture of two people; one was pushing down on the other's head and appearing to be dominating and controlling him. The picture was shown to a group of doctors who were asked how this might illustrate the relationship between doctors and managers. The doctors unanimously agreed that they were the underdogs and the management were in charge. The perception from the other side provided an interesting point of learning. The same picture was shown to a group of NHS managers. They were asked exactly the same question. The managers unanimously agreed that the doctors had all the power.

When we consider hierarchy, it is important to consider the *perceived* power differential. The perception in each group cited above was obviously very different.

Hierarchy is not standardized within an organization; there are micro-cultures and the gradients between groups can be very different. The culture in each micro-culture is strongly influenced by the personalities of individuals. People will ask 'who is on today?' knowing that this will affect whether they are going to have a 'good' day. Hierarchy, in simple terms, is a balance between the approachability of the leader and the assertiveness of the followers. Have you asked yourself whether people would stand by and watch you make a mistake, unable to find the words to challenge you? Have you asked them how approachable you are and what sort of leadership style they perceive that you use? If they answer too quickly or find either the floor or the ceiling suddenly interesting or tell you it is 'fine', I suggest some self-reflection might be worthwhile!

Some questions to ponder about your human interactions

How does your personal Myers–Briggs type indicator (MBTI), preferred learning style, and preferred team role affect those around you? Have you spent time analysing any tricky relationships that you have at work with those tools in mind? How good are you at adapting your style to meet the needs of others?

Have you mastered different ways to lead that have replaced 'pace-setting' (micro-management with a dictatorial time frame) and 'command and control'?

Have you mastered the coaching style that we know is currently used only by a handful of leaders across the NHS and yet will empower and achieve results? Or are you still making excuses that you 'don't have time for all of that' as you have to hit a target, etc?

Have you invested adequately in teaching and delegating?

We aim to develop a sense of trust in a team where everyone knows his or her role and he or she will do the right thing whether someone is watching or not. This approach has two advantages: it frees the leader up to be doing something else as he or she are no longer trying to micro-manage the team, and it allows the team to take responsibility, to use its own initiative and to develop.

Does your team feel like you trust each other? Or is the culture that is generated one where team members have to cover their backs?

How is your hierarchy? Would your team think it is the magical 15 degrees (see Level One, p. 60)? Have you asked? Have you asked your team what they think about your leadership style? Have you asked them how it could be improved?

When interacting with patients or staff have you become aware of your body language? Do you ever looked rushed? Do you let your patients see that? Have you altered your ward rounds, for example, so that it does not involve large numbers of people towering over someone's bed when the patient is in her nightwear?

Environment

We have highlighted how *where* we are influences how we think and what we might be expecting. For example, if I am working in a routine day-case theatre where all the patients are fit and healthy, then I may be less likely to be 'expecting the unexpected'. When it does happen, it may take me longer to perceive those changes and longer to act on them. If I am called to the emergency department, however, I go there with a slight adrenaline rush and I am already asking the question, 'what will the unexpected be?'

This is the first aspect of the triad of situation awareness, 'What?' 'So what?' 'What next?'

I use the analogy of a children's programme from my childhood. The main character was a scarecrow that could change his head to suit the occasion. We could substitute his changing heads with the term 'mindset'. If I am in routine day-case mode where I have done this procedure hundreds of times before, how can I make sure that I am error-aware and not complacent? Try to encourage your 'routine head' to stay curious: where might today's error spring from?

However, the environment contains many other influencing factors other than those which affect our expectations. The next is the familiarity. It is obviously useful to know where things are because if I need them in a hurry I can find them. Lack of familiarity with the environment is something commonly ticked on the SHEEP sheet.

Things would be very different if I am not at work but in a supermarket in 'mummy mode' when someone collapses in front of me. I have never planned in detail how I would manage an emergency in that environment. The same was true when I stopped to help someone on a rainy night on a road and I ended up helping in the back of an ambulance. Dealing with the same emergency on a ward is different from being in a clinic or a GP surgery, which is different from being in theatre, which is different from being in a corridor or a lift, which is different from being in a moving ambulance, which is different from being in someone's home, and so on.

How good are your induction programmes at orientating people to their environments? If you work somewhere new, how long do you spending familiarizing yourself with where everything is?

Think also of the environment's design. There are two aspects to this: first, the physical space of the walls and the immoveable objects over which we have no control (unless you are lucky enough to have input into a new build). We can, however, influence the use of that space: where things are stored, the position of things, and optimization and standardization of this storage. There are some very positive ideas on this in the 'productive' series (for more on this series, please see <http://www.institute.nhs.uk>).

The idea is to make it easy to do the right thing. Objects can be stored in groups that are associated with a task, e.g. urinary catheterization. Instead of having to hunt for the items, they are stored in a standardized way across the organization and perhaps one day even across different organizations. This would make errors when rotating jobs less likely as well as improving efficiency. If all the items I need for a task are presented to me in a logical way, I am more likely to use them than if I had to track them all down in separate places.

Some questions to ponder about your environment

How well organized is your environment? Have you standardized areas that have the same function?

What is your induction programme like for new starters with regards to where things are? Do you show them the things they really need to see? How do you know what they really need to see? Have you checked with them that they have seen them?

How will you stop yourself from becoming complacent in a routine situation?

How will you cope in an unexpected situation in an unexpected place?

I attended the collapse of someone in a supermarket, and waiting for the paramedics to arrive was struck with how alone I was without the team and equipment that I am used to having around me!

Equipment

I tend to categorize these very broadly into administrative and medical equipment.

We are increasingly dependent on our IT systems. Each organization seems to be developing its own system. This is not in keeping with the idea that standardization is the safer option. This leaves us with very large holes in the cheese at times of junior doctor handover—beware particularly in August and February (see Box 1.1)!

Box 1.1 Soap-box moment

I see this lack of standardization as a system error where the NHS is no longer one single organization but is being pushed to become competing mini-organizations. I think we should be very cautious of the safety implications of this approach. The loss of shared learning and each organization reinventing its own wheel is not the best way forward.

If we think about the medical equipment, the subject of standardization crops up again (see Example 1.3). Have we purchased one type of kit to perform one task, or do we have to learn to do it in lots of different ways using lots of different types of equipment?

Are all pieces of kit compatible with each other?

Example 1.3 Equipment example

If I move a critical patient from one area of the hospital to another, does the monitoring equipment look the same in each area? Am I expected to be able to process the information from completely different screens? Is it a waveform or numerical data? If I am relying on pattern recognition of a waveform to identify an arrhythmia (abnormal heart rhythm) or altered CO_2 trace (gas that we breathe out that helps us guide how well we are ventilating a patient or how well someone is breathing), is the waveform speed the same on different types of equipment? Are the same colours representing the same information? Is there a national standard? (The answer here is no, not yet!) Are the buttons the same or the menu options? If I have never seen the equipment before, will it be so intuitive that I can work out how to use it myself? Can I troubleshoot if necessary, by myself?

A few thoughts to ponder about equipment

How reliable is the equipment? Is it fit for purpose? Who checks that it is?

How is it maintained?

Did the last person who used it put it away broken or fail to wipe the blood off it? How and where is it stored? Is it easy to find?

Do you have enough of it?

Do your staff know how to use it? How do you know? What if it is only used rarely in an emergency setting? Do staff practice using it, just in case they need to do so, even if only rarely?

How do you know they haven't left anything inside someone at the end of a case? How sure are you of your checking system? What could make that go wrong?

How many ways could the patient receive the wrong blood product in your organization? Where are the hot spots and why?

Personal
Self-awareness

It is helpful during any high-pressure interaction to be able to master the 'balcony and dance floor' concept.[2] In the middle of events this involves taking a brief moment to imagine climbing above the situation as though climbing onto the balcony and having a look down at what is happening on the dance floor, including looking at oneself.

The self-assessment that needs to take place should cover a number of issues: stress levels, fatigue, cognitive workload, the effects of time pressure, team interactions, and a 'swan' assessment. I will start with the latter. The metaphor is a common one: it is used to explain the concept of looking calm and serene above the surface whilst underneath the feet are paddling like mad. When I ask how in touch someone is with their inner swan, I mean how good are they at giving an external appearance of calm no matter what is going on inside. The team needs the team leader to be a good swan and the leader needs this too from his or her followers.

We will cover other concepts in more depth in later chapters, but as a starting point it is sufficient to know that being tired can impairment judgement as much as consuming alcohol. High stress levels, time pressures, and high cognitive workload (having to think about lots of things at once) commonly contribute to making errors.

A simple way of keeping everyone up to speed with what you are thinking which serves the dual purpose of keeping your own stress levels at bay is something called **commentating**. For those of you who have ever watched police chases on television, you will have witnessed this activity as police describe the route they are taking out loud. Using this technique is extremely useful at many levels: your team can follow the direction you are taking (allows the shared mental model to develop, and it helps streamlines your thoughts, blocking out the multiple trains of thoughts that try to surface during high-cognitive workload, moments of high stress, and it acts almost as a filtering mechanism).

If in doubt, go back to basics. In an emergency setting that might mean default to ABC (airway, breathing, circulation). In a non-clinical setting that might mean 'let's summarize what we know so far, who is doing what, and where we need to get to'.

High stress levels not only have an effect on the way our thoughts are processed and decisions made, but affect our manual dexterity. I heard a metaphor recently which I think is particularly apt: the 'boxing gloves of stress'. It is these *boxing gloves* that convert the easy cannulation or blood taking into a 'difficult venous access', the straightforward intubation into a 'difficult airway', the dental extraction into something far more challenging than expected. Getting the projector and laptop to work together at the beginning of a speech is so much harder because you are being watched. Can you make a mental list of what triggers your stress levels to rise? Common ones include unfamiliar environment, unfamiliar team, unusual procedure or patient group, time pressure or high workload, high background stress level due to life events, fatigue, and anything that moves you outside of your comfort zone.

So in essence, we are asking how can we keep a clear head and remove our boxing gloves in a situation that we find stressful? The techniques that we discussed in Level One to rein in the physiological stress response were the NASA two-breath technique or the martial arts-derived 'in for 7, out for 11'. To add to these is the 'square' technique. Find a square that you can see or visualize one. Breathe in as you go along one side and breathe out as you go along the next, in as you go along the third side, and out as you go along the fourth. ('Go along' could mean trace it with your finger, follow it with your eyes, or imagine doing so.) Any of these techniques breaks the cycle of racing thoughts, temporarily replaces them with a task that requires focus, and then allows the thoughts to be regrouped. Being aware of your own stress levels is the first step; learning to manage them and intervene is the next part to master.

Knowing your limitations is also vital. It is not a sign of failure to ask for help; it is an essential part of patient safety. The trainees that I am most concerned about are those that have an over-inflated view of their own abilities. However, this is also true for consultants or any person in a senior role. There is no magical moment when we progress up the ladder that suddenly makes us able to know and do everything. (I admit when I was a medical student, I was under this illusion, that one day I would just know all the answers. However, as I became older I realized that there is a lot less black and white and a lot more grey!) What age has given me is the experience to cope with this ambiguity.

If you are one of those more senior professionals, do you still ask for help? When was the last time you worked alongside some of your colleagues and you gave each other some peer review? Have you ever struggled on longer than you should have? Who could you call next time for some advice? There is a quotation about swallowing one's pride as it is not fattening, which I rather like.

This ability to show vulnerability at the top leads me back to the topic of hierarchy, which we have already discussed.

Early results from the SHEEP sheet

The earliest results from the SHEEP sheet seem to indicate that the most common sources of error are factors in the human interaction and personal sections. Not surprisingly, top of the current list is a problem with communication alongside high workload and time pressure. Frustration, tiredness, and interruptions are the next most-cited reasons on the list. Lack of familiarity with a guideline, personality clashes, attitudes, temperature, noise levels, along with hunger, thirst, and stress are in the next frequency category. I emphasize that these results are provisional but we should have enough data to draw meaningful conclusions soon.

Key points

♦ SHEEP stands for Systems, Human Interaction, Environment, Equipment, Personal

Systems

♦ By changing how we approach error, we can use our knowledge of the SHEEP sheet factors to identify high-risk days and then put in extra steps to try to prevent the error

- By using a briefing/debriefing sandwich as part of regular working we can identify errors before they happen and ensure continual learning if they have occurred

- Lots of learning can happen from unpicking why a day went well

- We need better systems of promoting organizational learning both within an organization and across organizations

Human interaction

- Good morale can affect on outcome in terms of both mortality and morbidity: ban the 'Mood Hoover'

- Problems with communication or information flow are a major contributory factor to error

- Read back, cross check, active identification, and open questioning should be techniques familiar to all healthcare professionals no matter what their grade or profession

- The generic non-technical skills framework (G-NO-TECS) can be used to help teams examine how they work together

Environment and equipment

- We would benefit from standardization of both environments and equipment. Legislation to encourage manufacturers to conform cannot come soon enough.

- We need to place more emphasis on design, familiarity, and standardization of both our equipment and our environment

Personal

- Self-awareness of stress levels, cognitive workload, fatigue, and ability are a vital component of safety

References

1. Buttigieg SC, West MA, Dawson JF. Well-structured teams and the buffering of hospital employees from stress. *Health Services Management Research A* 2011; 24(4): 203–12.
2. Heifetz R. *Leadership Without Easy Answers*. Cambridge, MA: Belknap Press of Harvard University Press, 1994.

2

Situational awareness

'The true art of memory is the art of attention.'
Samuel Johnson
1709–84

Introduction

For me, the simplest way to consider this concept is Endsley's[1] *'what, so what, what next?'* This allows us to look at the three processes that contribute to situational awareness: *perception* of what is going on around us, making sense of that perception or *comprehension* and what that means for the *current state*, and then the *projection to the future state* and its implications. We will consider each of these in turn and introduce some practical examples.

We will consider what factors may impair our situational awareness, why we should worry about it, and apply this knowledge to look at what techniques we might employ to improve situational awareness and maintain it.

Perception

The *Concise Oxford Dictionary* definition is:

1. The ability to see, hear, or become aware of something through the senses.

2. A way of regarding, understanding, or interpreting something.

(Reproduced with permission from the Concise Oxford English Dictionary, 12th edition. Copyright © 2011 Oxford University Press, Oxford.)

The senses that are going to be important for perception in the context of situational awareness in a healthcare setting are visual (body language, facial expression, physical signs of illness; for example, you may detect a rash or an altered gait; notice who else is in the room and whether or not you know them, and what roles they are fulfilling, where you are, what the monitor says; decipher an illegible entry in the notes; interpret a chest X-ray; digest a lengthy policy document or report, or a long list of blood results or a spreadsheet of financial data), auditory (you may hear what people are saying: patients, relatives, staff, a patient call-bell, background noise, the regular beep of a monitor with a heart rate, an alarm to tell you the parameter is abnormal, the noise of a diathermy machine, the telephone or a bleep), and sometimes touch (the 'pop' as a cannula enters a vein, the feel of the bowel while operating, the palpation of an abdomen, the tone in a limb, the loss of resistance on finding the epidural space, the temperature of the skin when the patient is peripherally shut down, the feedback from a wire as it passes along the blood vessel unimpeded, the hardness of the 'lump', the crepitus in a joint, or the clammy handshake of an anxious patient) (see Figure 2.1).

At its simplest level, a signal travels from the sensory organ in question to a specialized area of the brain that receives those signals: visual, auditory, or sensory cortex. The next step is more complicated. The brain 'chooses' what to do with this information; should it be ignored or filtered or held in a waiting bay or stored or processed? How we choose to handle this information depends on what else is going on in our brain at the time.

Part of this 'choosing' whether we actually perceive information is to do with our **attention**. If we are paying attention to one task and we are focused on it, something else can happen right in front of us and we won't see it (inattentional blindness).

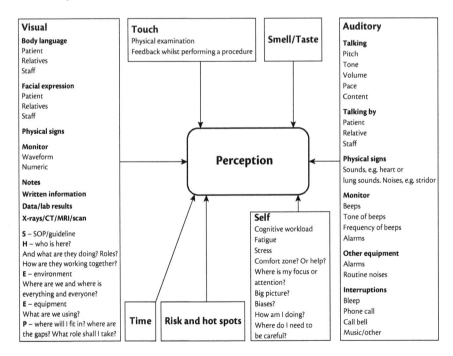

Figure 2.1 Perception inputs to situational awareness.

As far as visual processing goes, it is fairly easy to confuse our brains into thinking we have seen something that isn't really there or for us to miss something that is right under our nose because the focus of our attention is elsewhere.

There are plenty of examples of visual illusions on the Internet to help you explore this if you need convincing of these facts. (For an example, see: <http://brainden.com/face-illusions.htm#prettyPhoto>).

The effect of focusing on or attending to one task and missing something else can also be explored (See <https://www.youtube.com/watch?v=yrqrkihlw-s>; this clip will also explain my reference earlier in the book to a gorilla or moon-walking bear.)

This may all be very interesting and even a bit of fun, but what has it got to do with healthcare?

One of the key points is that we generally see what we expect to see. There are two types of bias that are relevant to this issue, expectation bias and confirmation bias. (In total there are currently thought to be about 150 different types of cognitive bias.)

If I hold out an ampoule of drug and ask you to check it I can influence what you see by telling you what it is; this was covered in Chapter 1. This is the reason that the cross check has to be performed accurately (see Box 2.1).

Box 2.1 Confirmation bias examples and cross check

Just a bit of revision on how to do a cross check.

I should *always* ask you, 'What is this?'

I should *not* say, 'lignocaine 1 per cent' (the ampoule in my hand is actually 2 per cent, as someone had 'tidied up' and put the ampoule back in the wrong box). I should *not* say 'amoxicillin' as I read the name on the ampoule (as actually this ampoule was next to amiodarone on the shelf and I have picked up the wrong drug). I should *not* say, 'this is a size-x lens' (when the stocking system seemed to have gone awry and this lens is not the size I thought I was selecting). I should *not* say, 'this is a right knee replacement ...' (when I have accidentally selected a left one).

In each case, I should simply be asking, '*what is this*?'

By telling you what you will see, I am introducing confirmation bias. You are much less likely to spot my error if I ask you to agree with me.

This will also be influenced by who we are, how well we know each other, whether you trust me, whether I am senior to you or respected or perhaps even a bit of a hero in the department, how much time pressure we are under, whether we are interrupted, what other things we are trying to do concurrently, whether we are tired, background noise levels, lighting levels, whether we have done the task so many times together that we have become complacent, and so on.

Another example of confirmation bias can be found in Level One where a liver biopsy was performed on the wrong patient. The doctors asked the person in bed, 'Mrs Brown?' Although the woman was not called Mrs Brown, she nodded in agreement. If two doctors arrive at your bedside, you might not really take in what they are saying nor think clearly and hence you may simply agree with them—bias number one. The doctors assumed it was Mrs Brown as the woman was in Mrs Brown's bed. They saw what they expected to see—bias number two. These two biases led to the death of the patient.

However, errors of perception do not occur solely in connection with drugs and procedures; perception errors are also relevant to making a diagnosis, clinical reasoning, non-clinical problem solving, and decision making (see Examples 2.1, 2.2, and 2.3).

Example 2.1 Dr X is my hero

If at handover we have been told that the diagnosis is acute asthma, do we *make an assumption* that the diagnosis is correct? When we meet the patient, do we make sure that this diagnosis fits what we perceive the history *and* signs *and* symptoms *and* observations *and* results might tell us? *Or* do we simply start with the diagnosis and fit what we perceive around the diagnosis?

What happens if new information becomes available that suggests the shortness of breath may be from another cause and actually there is a degree of heart failure, how good are we at questioning the original diagnosis?

Thinking but not verbalized: 'I don't think I can hear wheeze, it sounds more like fine creps to me ... but I'm just the ... junior/student/nurse. Surely Dr X would know. He's very senior. It must be my ears.'

Example 2.2 Changing a misdiagnosis

Patient Y was admitted three days ago. A well-respected middle-grade doctor made the diagnosis for patient Y. Since then there have been six shifts of nursing staff and the patient has been reviewed by doctors of all grades seven times. The working diagnosis has been passed on at each handover and it has never been challenged. New test results have arrived back that do not fit the original diagnosis, but still the shared mental model is the initial one that was made.

No-one has asked the questions 'what else could this be? How does this new information alter our original mental model and hence our decision making?'

In addition, the patient's routine medication was not prescribed. Everyone assumed that this was done on admission and so no-one looked for this. It is difficult to perceive an omission. If you simply look at the drug chart, how will you know something is missing? To find an omission you need to check two lots of information against each other: what is the patient's routine medication, does this match what has been prescribed, and then, has it been administered correctly since admission?

You will only see what you are looking for.

Patient Y collapsed on day 3. Only then were both the diagnosis re-examined and the drug chart reviewed adequately to spot the omissions.

We need a system that does not allow us to wait until a crisis occurs but instead tries to prevent it from happening. We need to stay curious.

Could the working diagnosis be wrong?

What could we have missed?

Does any new information alter our working diagnosis?

Example 2.3 Mrs B

I return to the death of my friend Mrs B from Level One.

At medical school I was told that 'common things are common' as part of my training in diagnostics. At a population level this concept may indeed be true but I think this attitude can be hazardous when applied to an individual.

When someone in their mid-forties presents with urinary symptoms, the commonest diagnosis may well be a urinary-tract infection. However, at what point do we change that thinking or mental model? After how many repeated admissions should we seek more extensive tests? If we do not ask the right question—'how many times has this happened?'—how will we get the right answers?

I say again:

Could the working diagnosis be wrong?

What could we have missed?

Does any new information alter our working diagnosis?

I will always wonder whether these questions could have saved my friend's life.

There are three more aspects to consider within this section that are very important in the healthcare setting: perception of the passage of time, the perception of risk, and the avoidance of task-fixation error.

Perceiving the passage of time

> *The distinction between past, present and future is only an illusion, however persistent.*
>   Albert Einstein, 1879–1955

In Level One, we talked about how, when our cognitive workload is high, it is very easy to lose track of how much time has elapsed. Think, for example, of trying to obtain venous access in a neonate, extracting a tricky molar, negotiating an endoscope around a corner where it just doesn't want to go, struggling with a hot gall bladder that is incredibly stuck down, trying to locate an epidural space in someone with a high body-mass index who is contracting very frequently, persuading the wire to bend up into a vessel at a tricky angle, running a trauma resuscitation with a team of eight people at the bedside of a young person who was hit by a drunk driver and so you just 'have to get them back', or reading a long list and you realize you have forgotten what was at the beginning: what was the first example I used in this list? Don't peek!

It all comes back to where our attention is focused. If we focus on the task, we lose track of time.

We have already identified 'loss of sense of time' as posing a risk in an acute setting, and we have talked about the 'antidote'—allocating this role to a member of the team. This team member, the **time keeper**, calls out time checks and relevant other observations. The time keeper focuses his or her attention only on time keeping and time checks (verbalizing the time *and* making sure that this is heard. This is best achieved with read back or closed-loop communication). See Example 2.4.

> ## Example 2.4 Time check with closed-loop communication
>
> In a cardiac-arrest setting, the cycles on the current guideline last for two minutes. The time keeper tells the team leader, possibly adding the team-leader's name to get his or her attention in the melee, 'we have reached two minutes'. The team leader acknowledges the information and repeats the time check to the whole team with an instruction of what the team is going to do next.
>
> 'Tim, we are at two minutes with this cycle,' says Alfie who is the time keeper.
>
> Tim acknowledges Alfie with a nod of the head, eye contact, and a thumbs-up to show that he has heard him. He gathers his thoughts, glances at the guideline as he is using his cognitive aid, and then addresses the group.
>
> 'We are at two minutes. Please continue cardiac massage until I say stop, then we will swap in a new person to take over the massage and do a rhythm assessment at the same time. Are you ready to swap in, Andrea? Darren, are you ready to do the rhythm check and pulse check if required? On my count …'.

This time keeper is a vital role in any acute setting. It is relatively easy to allocate someone to time keeping if you know it is an emergency, but what if this is a routine case that is becoming tricky?

What if what was a routine everyday thing that you do, is starting to deviate from the norm? How will you detect this change? The fact that it is taking longer than normal is a cue. But how will you maintain your perception of time?

How will you know that you have tried for long enough and that now you should call for help either from someone more senior or a fresh pair of eyes or a different skill set (see Exercise 2.1)?

Exercise 2.1 Identifying your 'hot spots', including loss of time perception and the 'sterile cockpit'

I would like you to grab a pen and a piece of paper: yes, really. You won't be able to do this in your head and I wonder how many of you just rolled your eyes?

We are going to build a table with four columns as illustrated in Table 2.1. The table will have four headings.

Table 2.1 Failure-mode effect analysis table to identify 'hot spots'

Activity step	Failure mode	Effects	Analysis

Column 1 is labelled *Activity step*.

To populate column 1, I want you to make a list. I would like the list to be written in a column going down the left-hand side of the page.

I would like you to start by thinking of any high-risk activities that you perform where if you get it wrong, serious harm may come to a patient or another member of staff.

I want you to choose one example of a high-risk activity from this mental list. I want you to break the activity down into a list of steps and write them in column 1. The more steps you can break it down into the better.

Remember that harm can also come from omitting a task (e.g. not relieving a pressure area, or missing a drug dose, or failing to identify a patient before a procedure), not just by carrying out the activity or procedure.

In column 1, I want you to name the step in the activity rather than the omission (for example, this could be 'pressure care', or 'drug administration', or 'patient identification').

Now think of an example of an activity that you perform that needs a lot of concentration or brain power (high cognitive workload).

Examples might include a difficult problem to solve, perhaps a task that has a lot of detail, lots of facts or figures, or perhaps one that is drug-related. Are there mathematical calculations that you need to perform? Are you juggling lots of activities all at once, or perhaps learning to do something new so you have to concentrate harder; it may be a tricky skill which requires a lot of dexterity; it may be a consultation or a meeting with a highly emotional content and you need to listen really hard and make sure you pick up all the cues; it may be that you are in an unfamiliar environment and so you don't know where anything is and this converts something usually routine into something more challenging.

Once you have thought of an example, break that activity down into steps and add the steps to column 1.

To summarize, in column 1 we should be trying to consider a high-risk activity, and an activity that has a high cognitive workload. Both of these two examples should be broken down into as many steps as possible. The steps should be listed in column 1.

During both of these types of activities we are at risk of losing track of time.

In column 2, which we are going to call *failure mode*, I would like you to say *how* each step of the activity could go wrong or fail.

For example, you could forget to do that particular step, or not complete that step accurately. You might use the wrong technique, or fail to follow a guideline, or you could take too long to complete the step so that it is delayed, for example, you could lose track of time or get distracted when someone interrupts you.

For now, just use one mode of failure for each step, but be aware that there may be a number of different ways in which each step could fail. Make sure you carefully consider whether loss of sense of time might be relevant to the step you are considering.

For example, if we think about the using a defibrillator, we could fail to follow the guidelines for safe defibrillation. If we are trying to intubate, we could lose track of time. If you are doing a drug round, someone might interrupt you.

In column 3, which we are going to call *effects*, I want you to write down what would happen if each step of the activity went wrong.

In the defibrillator example, if we don't make sure that everyone is 'clear', we may harm another member of staff when we shock them!

If we lose track of time while we are trying to intubate, we may render our patient hypoxic (low oxygen levels).

If someone interrupts you on a drug round, you may give out the wrong drug, or the wrong dose, or miss a drug dose, or give something to the wrong patient.

In column 4, which we will call *analysis*, I want you to write down a few thoughts about how serious a problem would be if it happened at this step.

I want you to try to look down the list and select which might be the most important steps or 'hot spots', as these would have the biggest impact if they went wrong.

I want you to choose these 'hot spots' and make them visible on your table. These are the ones we need to focus on first.

What safety features might you need to introduce?

Is there anything you could do more of in order to prevent this from happening, or anything you ought to do less of (for example, do we need to do more time checks and interrupt less)?

How can you make an awareness of the risks of a loss of sense of time be higher in your priorities? What measures will help?

Some of you will be familiar with the mini process that we have informally started here. It is a quick version of a failure mode and effects analysis (FMEA).

By focusing on the *hot spots* with our teams, we can ensure that the focus of their attention is on the 'at-risk' steps. You cannot expect to maintain a high level of attention continuously and neither can you expect this to be the sole solution to the problem, so it is important for the team to know which steps to really take seriously.

During the hot spots, it may be necessary that no-one talks unless it is essential for the procedure. This type of concept is sometimes referred to as the '*sterile cockpit*'. There should be no interruptions during this time.

No-one should be talking about what they are going to do at the weekend or what is the next case. It should be possible to identify some of these hot spots during a briefing or huddle when you meet up to plan the day. Some hot spots should be routine.

Routine hot spots for the benefit of the anaesthetist would include induction (when you are putting someone to sleep), emergence (when you are waking someone up), any time that you are drawing up a drug or working out a drug dose, and when you are transferring someone (either from the anaesthetic room to the operating theatre, or from the operating theatre to recovery), and then settling them into that new environment (e.g. attaching all the monitoring equipment to the patient's body).

We have already mentioned that all dispensing, preparation, and drug administration should be thought of as hot spots.

Patient identification should be a hot spot.

When are your routine hot spots?

Then there will be patient-specific and procedure-specific hot spots. For example, there may be a part of the surgery that is particularly challenging in the person with diabetes and a high BMI who needs a bowel resection. This could be identified at the briefing and then highlighted when the tricky part is about to start.

I hope doing this mini-FMEA and hot-spot identification will prompt you to do this exercise on a broader scale and give it a lot more thought.

Task-fixation error

So, playing devil's advocate, why is it that we have developed this ability to lose track of time and concentrate our attention on just one thing?

It can, of course, be vital to block out everything else around you so that you can focus on something difficult. For the type of task that we will discuss in Exercise 2.6, where we have a high cognitive workload, it is an obvious advantage for us not to be distracted by what is going on around us so we shut it out.

If we are working as part of a team and each team member focuses really hard on the aspect of the whole he or she is undertaking and performs it really well, there shouldn't be a problem as long as someone is maintaining an overview of all the individual tasks. In other words, we need a hands-off leader (i.e. only leading, not performing one of the tasks), like the conductor of an orchestra, keeping us to time and encouraging us all in the same overall direction.

If we do not have the luxury of having this many team members then we need to use a timer to monitor what we are doing, perhaps a machine that can beep at us when the time is up or a time-keeping team member, to help us avoid falling into this trap.

If you are a member of a team and you have been focusing hard on a task (for example, establishing venous access in a neonate with difficult veins) and you have now completed that task, you need to be aware of the need to *transition*. This is the ability to change from that focused state back to taking in everything around you again. To do this you may need to ask for a summary of the points that we can use to help with our situational awareness: *What? So what? What next?* (see Box 2.2 for the SHEEP adaptation of Endsley's[1] situational awareness).

Box 2.2 The SHEEP adaptation of Endsley's[1] situational awareness: SHEEP awareness

What?

What is the working diagnosis or *what* is the problem definition?

So what? (SHEEP)

So what management **plan/SOP** are we using? (S)

What staff are **doing what**? (H) How are we working together?

What place is most appropriate to be dealing with this episode? What influence might this have on people in other areas? (E)

What equipment are we using? (E)

What about me (how is my cognitive workload, how is my fatigue level, how full is my bucket, where is my focus, am I keeping track of time, do I need help?) (P)

What next? (SHEEP)

What else might we need to try *next*? Is there a SOP that might help? (S)

What other **staff** might we need? Who else might need to know about this? (H)

What environment is most suitable and does this involve us moving? (E)

What other **equipment** might we need soon? (E)

What about me (cognitive workload, fatigue, where is my focus, how long have we been going, will I need help as this unfolds?) (P)

Self-awareness: The perception phase

Part of our ability to maintain our situational awareness involves us maintaining our self-awareness.

The balcony and the dance floor

I find the Heifetz[2] metaphor of the 'balcony and the dance floor' helpful for this. Whenever we are interacting with someone else, be it in a group meeting, a one-to-one interaction, a consultation, a clinical encounter, or an emergency setting, the idea is that we maintain a balcony view of ourselves on the dance floor.

This may include asking questions from that balcony position, looking down at yourself and asking yourself 'what is my cognitive workload? Am I tired? How are my stress levels? Am I out of my depth? Do I need help?'

But it may include other questions about yourself: where is my attention? What could I be missing? How am I functioning within this team or in this interaction? Am I experiencing any emotions here that may be influencing the encounter? If so, what is triggering those emotions? Am I sharing my mental model adequately? How might my behaviour be influencing what is happening in this team? What might I need to alter?

Fatigue and stress: Personal perception

We have identified that being either tired or stressed can affect how we function, not only in how we perceive things, but how well we can perform cognitive processes, and how well we can perform physical tasks (the boxing gloves of stress, from Chapter 1). It is therefore important that you can identify both these states in yourself and then take the next step to put in measures to counteract them.

Step 1: When might you might be tired?

I would like you to think about your working week and identify any key times when you might be tired. Do you work nights? Do you change from nights to days? Is there a very heavy day in your week when you work a very long shift and you know you don't normally get a break? Do you care for children or a relative who needs you at night? Are you stressed and so not sleeping well?

Step 2: What does being tired feel like for you?

How do you know you are tired? What will it feel like for you? Do you have to wait until you are yawning? Can you feel your mental processing slowing down a bit? Are you a bit grumpy or impatient or less tolerant? Are your energy levels below normal? Are you aware that you can't concentrate as well? Can you multi-task less easily so you have to break things down a bit more into bite-sized chunks?

We will now repeat those questions for stress.

Step 1: What makes you feel stressed?

As part of getting to know ourselves it is useful to understand what 'presses our buttons'.

At the risk of seeming very intolerant I will share some of my own: a problem with the children before I leave for work, no cup of tea before I start, traffic jams and no car-parking space, a delayed train (I hate being late, other people being late or not turning up), laziness, rudeness, shouting, being asked to move the goalposts without any consideration of the extra time that may be involved, in fact time pressure in general, people showing others a lack of respect, power games, the list could go on. All of these are aggravated if I'm tired or hungry!

I need you to be aware of your equivalent list and to stay alert to your triggers throughout your working day.

Step 2: What does stress feel like for you?

How do you know you are becoming stressed?

When I ask this question of people on my courses, here are some of the replies I get: flushing of skin or turning red (often chest or neck or face), heart rate speeds up, aware of heart thumping, sweaty palms, headache, muscles tense, shoulders tense up, can't think straight, go quiet, talk incessantly, butterflies in the stomach, develop a short fuse, become intolerant, stop listening and 'on edge'.

Which combination of these might apply to you?

Team situational awareness: Perception

It is vital to consider the team approach to situational awareness because in healthcare settings when emergencies occur we should rarely be on our own for any length of time. If we are the first on scene, we need to think about where our help might be and how we will activate it. This is important in both a setting where emergencies happen regularly but, perhaps even more so, where they are rare and infrequent. Rehearsal or simulation of these emergencies is very useful as a dry run to test the system, not just for the benefit of the individuals involved. There are obvious advantages in an emergency setting to having a team approach where the individuals can simultaneously work at parallel tasks that contribute to the whole treatment plan. However, good team working is not a chance activity.

With a number of people working together there will be an opportunity to amalgamate the perceptions of multiple individuals. Each may bring a different perspective and different experience. The first challenge is how to ensure that people feel able to offer their ideas on both the cues they perceive and how they might interpret those cues (this is influenced by hierarchy, assertiveness, approachability of leader, presence of a hero figure, organizational culture, departmental micro-culture, experience, and team training).

The subsequent challenge is how these ideas are then coordinated to feed into a 'big picture' or mental model. We will cover this phase in the section on comprehension.

Of course, team working is not only important in the emergency setting. Team working is vital when making complex decisions that require multi-professional angles to optimize patient care. (Example 1, an MDT (multi-disciplinary team) working in cancer care to coordinate the optimum timing and combination of surgery, radiotherapy, and chemotherapy treatments).

The different perspectives offered by a broader team will make for much better decision making. (Example 2, for a patient with a complex chronic condition who will need integrated shared care between primary, secondary, and social care, the combined knowledge of these different groups will have far more to offer than one of the sectors in isolation.)

In both of these non-acute settings the principles are similar. It is still important that everyone feels that they have a voice, no matter what their professional background, and that there opinion is valued. The subsequent challenge is also a parallel one: how to coordinate these different perspectives to build towards a shared mental model or problem definition.

Perception: The story so far

We have established that it is easy for us to miss things. We have tried to look at times when we are more at risk of this happening. We have established that when we have a high cognitive work load, are tired or stressed, we are more at risk of missing something. We have identified some particular at-risk times during our work days and I hope you may introduce a 'sterile-cockpit' approach to these hot spots to help make perception and indeed comprehension easier. I hope you are going to consider ways to avoid the 'loss of time perception' trap.

After we have perceived what is going on, we then need to process it, make sense of it, and apply this knowledge to our work.

We need to consider the management plan (S), staffing (H), environment (E), equipment (E), and ourselves (P), and how to apply these to the situation that we face.

Comprehension and its implications for current state

Memory

Let us assume that we have paid enough attention to something that is going on around us so that we have indeed perceived it. We now have to make sense of what we have perceived and use that understanding to inform our current actions. (Incidentally, in the meantime, we need to continue perceiving!)

Our awareness will need to go beyond what we can see, hear, or touch.

In order to make sense of things we need to involve what we already have knowledge of and have experienced. We will need to evoke memory recall.

In addition to helping with our understanding of situational awareness, an understanding of how human memory can be fallible is useful. With this in mind we can then use a few practical steps to help ensure the safety of our patients (see Examples 2.5 and 2.6).

Example 2.5 Memory recall: The job list

If I ask you to do an ECG on Professor Plum in bed 1, a full blood count on Mr Scarlett in bed 7, and a 'U and E' on Colonel Mustard in bed 10, if I simply recited the list to you and you hadn't written it down, or done any read back, how likely do you think it would be that you would remember all the information accurately?

The general thoughts on how many things we can probably remember seem to be seven, plus or minus two.[3] I gave you nine pieces of information. Without re-reading them now, try to recall them now and count them on your fingers. How did you do?

If we tackle the information differently before we try to remember it, we stand a better chance of remembering it all. If we group the information into three groups of three, we are 'chunking' the information. We can also theme it. The names should ring bells as those in a popular board game (Plum, Scarlett, and Mustard), and they are also colours, and these details may help with our memory. There are three tests; ECG, full blood count, and U and E. There are three bed numbers; 1, 7, and 10.

I would like you to look away from the text for a moment and count to 15 slowly.

Now how many can you recall?

Whilst it may be easier this time, I hope that it emphasizes that all task lists should be written down and not left to chance!

Example 2.6 Remembering and talking to yourself

If I ask you to prepare a drug infusion for me, I would like you to read the instruction just once. I would like you to repeat the instruction to yourself over and over out loud for 30 seconds. Then I would like you to write it down and check it for accuracy.

Are you ready?

I would like 50 mg of drug B, made up to 50 mls with fluid P, to run at 5 mls an hour.

How did you do? By keep on repeating it you should be able to hold it repeatedly in your shorter term part of your memory. However, if you are interrupted during that process, the information will 'fall out' of your memory store and you will have to start again. If however, you have it in written form from the beginning you stand a better chance of reducing the error.

Now that we have explored the fallibility of human memory, we return to how we use our working memory and introduce the concept of capacity.

Capacity

At this point I'm going to introduce the concept of buckets (see Figure 2.2 for the SHEEP stress bucket). I want to imagine the capacity of our brain as a bucket that we can fill with 'stuff'. The amount of 'stuff' that we have already going on in our brains is what is already in the bucket: the tricky journey to work this morning, no car-parking space, the history and blood results of the six patients I have just seen this morning before the operating list, the agenda for the meeting at 5 p.m., the children's birthday party at the weekend, and the fact that we are nearly out of dog food. How full is your bucket?

If your bucket is already full, there is little brain capacity left for more cognitive processing.

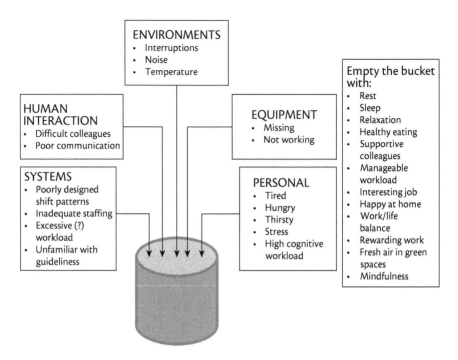

Figure 2.2 The SHEEP stress bucket.

There are two metaphors that I think are useful in this setting: multiple buckets or my scarecrow metaphor from Level One.

Using the first, imagine that you have many buckets and that you can empty your main bucket into these other buckets: perhaps an 'at-home' bucket, filled with the children's party and the dog food. Then perhaps another bucket: a 'not-relevant-now' bucket: tip the journey in, the car park, and the meeting into this one. This leaves only the six patients and the operating list for you to focus on. I have successfully reduced what is in your current bucket.

Using the second metaphor, imagine that you have more than one head and you can choose to put on the one for a given occasion. This would mean that the 'mummy' head, 'stressed driving in and car parking' head, and the 'meeting' head that you will need later are all removed, leaving just a clear 'six patients and an operating list' head.

Whichever method you adopt for **_transitioning or compartmentalizing_**, it is an important part of allowing enough of your cognitive capacity to be freed up for the comprehension phase of situational awareness.

Creating a mental model

Assuming that we have perceived something *and* we have some knowledge and possibly some experience we can draw upon *and* we can recall these from our memory *and* we have enough capacity in our bucket to process everything, we can start to think about how we make sense of it.

I think that how we build this mental model is strongly influenced by where we are in an organization (and by this I mean our physical location), and what we are expecting to see there. I am going to call this 'environmental bias'.

If we normally work in an acute area where emergencies are common and things are unplanned, I believe there is a 'filter question' that we ask almost simultaneously as we start to perceive. I think this question is something along the lines of, 'is this patient *sick*?' (and by *sick*, I mean seriously ill in a high-risk way), or 'is this life threatening?', or 'is this an emergency?' I believe if we dissect this filtering question we are actually asking two things—is this high risk and do we need to act quickly here?

If the answer, drawn from our very first perceptions is 'yes' then we start a different process than if we are facing something more routine.

I want you to imagine that you are approaching a patient in the 'resus bay' of a hospital (the resuscitation bay, an area in the emergency department where the sickest patients come in). What cues would you look for to start deciding whether this is an emergency or establishing just how sick the patient might be? Assume you are walking towards the patient but are still at least 10 feet away. What if there are lots of staff around the bed? What if they look concerned? What if they all look busy attaching monitors and putting in drips? What if they are bringing over the crash trolley? What if the patient is lying flat and not moving? What if you can see lots of blood?

What have you picked up or perceived so far? What are you already thinking about? Has your heart rate increased ever so slightly?

I now want you to consider a completely different scene. Let us imagine an outpatient clinic, or a GP surgery, or a dental clinic waiting room. If you are asked to collect a patient from this waiting area and escort him or her to a consultation room, what are your thoughts now? If the patient is seated in the waiting room, chatting to a relative and, after your active identification to ensure that you have collected the correct patient, he stands unaided and is willing to walk with you to the room?

What are your first thoughts now? Are you asking yourself whether this is an emergency or have you already discounted the need for a first question as this in no way seems life threatening? How fast did that 'decision making' happen? Were you even aware of it? Have you, in fact, already done a mini-risk assessment?

Have you considered time pressure in this situation? Whilst there may be a time pressure from the clinic being over-booked and the fact that you are already running late, this time pressure is different from the time pressure of thinking the person in front of you might die unless you act quickly.

I am 'assuming' that in both of these examples it is relatively easy and quick to perceive differences in the situations. The comprehension phase in each of them involves successfully doing a mini-risk assessment that is sufficient to activate different decision-making pathways (decision making will be explored in detail in Chapter 3). In the first example, I am *assuming* that you have perceived that this is a high-risk situation where decisions will need to be made and actions taken swiftly. In the second situation I am *assuming* that there is no immediate risk perceived and that the consultation will take place in a different way following different 'standard operating procedures' or approaches. In each of these examples the initial comprehension phase will have happened very quickly, I suspect without much conscious thought or cognition. I suspect for the experienced clinicians amongst you it will have happened on 'autopilot'.

(We will look at the advantages and also the dangers of autopilot in Chapter 3.)

Let us consider another situation, a third option that is perhaps somewhere between the two. Imagine that you are on a ward. You are approaching the bay at the end of the ward and you turn the corner to see six beds. Two of the patients are sitting up in chairs by the side of their beds, one patient is walking tentatively across the bay using a frame, one bed is empty, and two patients are in their beds. In the centre of the bay are a nurse and a drug trolley.

What are your initial impressions now?

On arrival at the third bed, you see that the patient is lying down, turned away from you. First impressions seem to lead you to think that they are asleep. When you call the patient by name there is no response. One of your colleagues, who has approached the bed on the other side, goes a bit closer and speaks loudly near the ear of Mr Banks, 'Mr Banks, can you hear me?' There is still no response. What are you thinking now? How are you starting to make sense of this situation? What are your next steps?

Outcome 1

As you roll Mr Banks over towards you, he opens his eyes and explains that he didn't have his hearing aide in place.

Outcome 2

As you roll Mr Banks over towards you, he appears to be breathing but unconscious.

I want you to consider your reactions to reading the two sentences with different outcomes. The comprehension of each option has completely different implications. What would you do next in each of the two settings?

You may be making a more detailed *situational assessment* that is the first step of decision making whilst simultaneously initiating a series of actions.

Team situational awareness: Comprehension

Once the mental model is generated it is important that it is shared with the team at a 'big-picture' level.

In an acute setting, there should be sufficient detail so that the team members understand how his or her role/task fits into the whole but not too much detail that it distracts from the task at hand or causes cognitive overload. This is less vital when time pressure is not an issue.

There should be regular phases where the mental model is reviewed in light of new information (e.g. change in condition, observations, new history available, or the investigation results are now available). The team need to be given the opportunity to contribute new perceptions and any new ideas that they may have about their understanding of the episode.

Errors in comprehension and building an incorrect mental model

Misperception can lead to the wrong mental model. If we *miss* cues altogether or there are dominant cues that distract us and are perhaps red herrings, we will end up with an incorrect mental model.

The next error that can occur concerns how we interpret the cues we have perceived. Here we are drawing on our memory to recall both knowledge and past experience. If we *misinterpret* cues or use the wrong pattern of recognition, we will *misdiagnose* and this will result in the establishment of an incorrect mental model. It may be that we choose to *ignore* cues if we are already expecting a particular mental model. This expectation bias is dependent on both your environment (what you expect to see *there*) and past experience (what happened when you saw something similar).

While building a mental model, we can *falsely identify the true risk or seriousness* of the situation and we can *misjudge the time* available.

Another source of error in a mental model is a *failure to update* it as new information becomes available. This can fall into two broad groups: new information becomes available that tells us our original mental model was wrong and needs changing, or the condition can change and what was originally a stable patient, with a mental model of stable patient attached, is no longer up to date or valid as the patient has deteriorated.

Team-related situational-awareness errors

There are a couple of aspects to mention with regards to thinking as a group. One is that moods can spread and influence other members of the group. This can be positive or negative. In a positive sense it may help if, in a crisis situation, the leader maintains his or her swan and doesn't give off a vibe of panic! But the flip side can be falsely reassuring—group settings tend to make everyone feel comfortable and so intervention may not occur as quickly as it should ('they don't seem worried so I shouldn't be either').

There are also the dangers of assuming that we know what others are thinking and what they have or have not done. Chapter 1 touched on the fact that we are less likely to find fault with our hero or the actions he or she takes or the decisions that he or she might make.

The impression is of a linear process but of course reality is much more complex (see Figure 2.3). Whilst our focus moves from perception to comprehension and building a mental model, we must also to continue to perceive changes and cues. We need to update our mental model with this new information continually. We need to

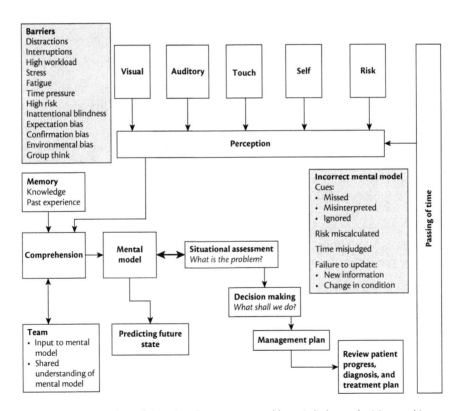

Figure 2.3 Overview of situational awareness and how it links to decision making.

keep assessing both whether the treatment is working and whether the baseline is changing at the same time.

In order to enhance our mental model it is important to gather input and ideas from our team. This should happen at each level: perception, comprehension, and mental model.

An example of how this might be achieved is given here first generically and then in a specific example taken from real life (Example 2.7).

There is an update and summary phase of gathering information from the team (including an update on observations, any new history or signs or symptoms present, or any more results available, or a pattern of these that are emerging that present themselves as a new cue). There can be a summary phase where the leader goes over all the cues that have been gathered so far and commentates on their thought processes that have led to the current mental model (or working diagnosis). The group/team are asked specific questions: 'What else could this be? What are we missing here? Are there any other staff/kit/tests that we should think about?' This process links to group decision making that will be covered in Chapter 3.

Example 2.7 Creating a shared mental model

Ward example. 33-year-old patient with known severe asthma. Previously ventilated on ICU. Suddenly collapsed in their bed. Unconscious but not arrested. Crash call went out. A team of seven is now in attendance at the bedside. We are coming to the scene after 15 minutes. The people in the team have introduced themselves and their roles have been clarified. There is an experienced and respected team leader agreed upon.

Leader: 'Ok. I'm going to come to each of you in turn so we can see how we are doing. Let's start at the top end. Airway—we have a size 7 tube in at 20 cm at the lips. Are we happy with that?'

Eye contact made and a 'yes, happy' response.

'Breathing—can we have another listen?' (Non-verbal communication as to who should listen). 'How easy is she to bag now?' (This comment is directed to the person with the bag, non-verbally).

'Still tight, maybe slightly easier since the magnesium.'

'Air entry improved since last time but still very quiet.'

Leader continues: 'Let's review the obs at this stage, and Julia, can you get ready to do another gas? Sats steady at 93 per cent, better end tidal CO_2 waveform.'

'Cardiovascular; how are we doing with that art line?'

Reply from someone kneeling by the bedside next to the patient's wrist: 'Just calibrating it now.'

'Perfect timing for that gas!'

'OK, heart rate 119, looks sinus. BP 145/89. What are we doing about sedation?'

The reply comes back that both infusions are being drawn up and it is agreed to give a dose of something else in the meantime. The gas is taken and sent straight to the nearest gas machine that is two wards away.

The leader asks the time keeper, who is documenting everything: 'Can you summarize how long we have been going and what we have given so far?'

'Anything else that we haven't mentioned?'

'So, we have A.B. who is a 33-year old with asthma who looks to have had a sudden deterioration today. We have started treatment for an acute episode of asthma. We have the guidelines here in front of us. Is there anything else we should be trying?'

A couple of ideas are floated. These suggestions are rewarded and encouraged.

'She has slightly improved from 10 minutes ago.'

'Any thoughts on why this might have happened?' Waits for replies and listens actively to each team member ensuring an opportunity for everyone to speak.

'Have we contacted her team?'

Team reply.

'Is there anyone else who might be able to help us with more information?'

Team offer up ideas.

This continues to cover the EEP of SHEEP.

I cannot emphasize enough that we also need to be aware that the situation will evolve over time and we need to be aware of what these future states may entail and how we might need to plan for them.

Failure to update a mental model in the light of new information is a recurrent healthcare error. We get stuck with our first mental model and it is hard to encourage people to move on to another perspective.

Predicting future state

As part of our current state assessment there also needs to be an understanding of whether we are keeping up with and, therefore, maintaining the status quo, or whether we are making progress or things are deteriorating.

This comprehension from a longitudinal point of view (i.e. how is the current state changing with time?) helps us to try to predict what we might need to next.

Acute/emergency setting/clinical/future-state prediction

I think we should always develop three plans. I am going to use a traffic light analogy.

Green option: If things improve

S—which treatment plan shall we follow now and in the short and the longer term?

H—which staff do we need and who should be doing what?

E—where do we need to be and how will we get there? (e.g. move to a ward from the emergency department, transfer from theatre to recovery, move from primary- to secondary-care setting)

E—what kit do we need?

P—hopefully my bucket will be less full! Can I get a micro-break to recover from this? When did I last eat/drink/empty my bladder?

How often will we reassess?

Amber option: We manage to maintain the current state

S—the current plan seems to be working; is there anything we can do improve on it? What might we be missing?

H—is there any additional expertise that would help us to improve things?

E—is there somewhere else we should be? (higher dependency level, investigation needed (e.g. CT scan), operating theatre, a more specialist hospital, transfer from primary to secondary care), and how would we get there?

E—is there additional more specialist equipment that would help us?

P—how full is my bucket? Am I still in my comfort zone? Would fresh eyes or additional expertise help? How often will we reassess? (Who is time keeping? Who will reassess?)

Red option: Things are continuing to deteriorate

S—the current treatment plan isn't working. What else could this be? What are we missing here? What else could we try?

H—have we got enough people here? Are they able to do the task they are allocated? Who else could help us?

E—can we move to a better place with more appropriate expertise? Is the patient stable enough to move? Or do we need the expertise to come here?

E—is there anymore kit that would help us? Do we need more tests or monitoring to give us more information about what we are dealing with?

P—I need to contact someone with more expertise if possible or run this by one of my peers if no-one more senior exists (e.g. you are the consultant). Is there another specialty that ought to be involved? Are my stress levels controlled? Am I commentating to ensure we have a shared mental model? Have I gathered thoughts and ideas from my team?

Has anything changed? How often are we reassessing? How much time has elapsed?

Can we pause, reassess now, and summarize where we are?

We are not the only sector who has to deal with emergencies regularly. I want to share with you the words used by the lead when fighting fires (I am regularly told by healthcare workers that we are fire-fighting, and so I hope the comparison is a useful one). The lead firefighter's name was Paul Gleeson and the work was publicized by Weike (Box 2.3).[4] Along with Sutcliffe, Weike has focused on assessing high-reliability organizations.

Box 2.3 Weick[4] quotes Gleeson

- Here's what I think we face
- Here's what I think we should do and why
- Here's what I think we should keep an eye on
- Now talk to me

If we look at 'future planning' we can do this with Gleeson in mind.

This future plan could be documented on a sheet of A4 as per Figure 2.4, and offers a tabular way you could quickly map out the three options for the future state.

Predicting future state: Routine clinical

When we see someone for a clinic visit in either an outpatient or a primary-care setting, predicting a future state requires a different framework.

In this setting one can take a more long-term view. It is not about how the condition will evolve in a matter of minutes or hours but instead perhaps how both the disease process and treatment will both impact on a future state of the individual which now may be weeks, months, or years ahead. It may even have implications for future generations. It could involve whether, for example, there will be implications for schooling, self-caring, needing more tests, or requiring surgery.

During this time frame, when the process of disease and treatment may both be changing, the clinician will not be present to observe it. It will, in fact, be the patient him or herself or perhaps a relative that will need to monitor and review progress in the interim. It may be important that we highlight to the patient what it is that he or she should be 'aware' of as this future state emerges. The patient will need to understand any particular issues that he or she needs to look out for following consultation. These changes in symptoms might be obvious to a healthcare professional but unless they are named explicitly, the patient may not know that they are important.

A firm plan needs to be in place agreed by both the patient and the clinician so that they have a shared mental model of the plan for both the treatment and the review process with clear timescales agreed. It should also be made clear, if things change from their expected course, what action should be taken. To achieve this adequately will involve robust communication skills ensuring clear explanations, read back, and clarification (see Figures 7.5 and 7.6 in Level One). The pitfalls of assumption will need to be avoided.

The sharing of this plan between different organizations (primary, secondary, and social care) should also be considered as part of this future state planning.

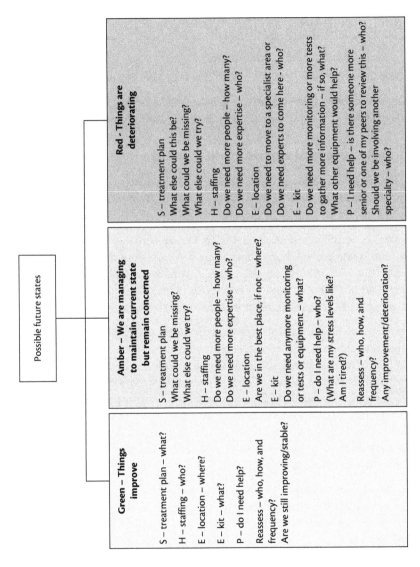

Possible future states

Green – Things improve

S – treatment plan – what?

H – staffing – who?

E – location – where?

E – kit – what?

P – do I need help?

Reassess – who, how, and frequency?
Are we still improving/stable?

Amber – We are managing to maintain current state but remain concerned

S – treatment plan
What could we be missing?
What else could we try?

H – staffing
Do we need more people – how many?
Do we need more expertise – who?

E – location
Are we in the best place, if not – where?

E – kit
Do we need anymore monitoring or tests or equipment – what?

P – do I need help – who?
(What are my stress levels like?
Am I tired?)

Reassess – who, how, and frequency?
Any improvement/deterioration?

Red – Things are deteriorating

S – treatment plan
What else could this be?
What could we be missing?
What else could we try?

H – staffing
Do we need more people – how many?
Do we need more expertise – who?

E – location
Do we need to move to a specialist area or
Do we need experts to come here – who?

E – kit
Do we need more monitoring or more tests to gather more information – if so, what?
What other equipment would help?

P – I need help – is there someone more senior or one of my peers to review this – who?
Should we be involving another specialty – who?

Figure 2.4 A template for the traffic-light approach to future state—green, amber, red SHEEP awareness

Future-state planning: Intermediate, clinical

There are, of course, many situations that do not fit into either the emergency or the routine categories that I have just described. Let us consider an inpatient who is currently stable but perhaps has multiple morbidities (pre-existing conditions that could complicate the course of treatment). It may be that the current illness for which the patient has been admitted may cause a deterioration in some of the other underlying conditions from which he or she suffers. In this case planning for a future state may be quite complex. It may be necessary for the multi-disciplinary team to plan together for some 'what if' options in both the short and longer term.

In the short term there may be some key parameters named that should be observed and the frequency that they should be looked at defined. The plan should describe how often the patient will need reviewing and by whom, and what level of seniority might be appropriate. Investigations and monitoring might be necessary to make sure we are actively seeking any signs of deterioration. Some key things to watch for should be clearly described to raise awareness and make sure that the focus of attention is correctly aligned so that we don't miss something that is right under our noses. In general, we will only find what we are looking for.

In the longer term, different plans may need to be considered with regard to home help, care packages, daily activities, dependent relatives, or discharge planning. Being aware of how the current condition and its future projections impact on these things will feed into the decision-making processes.

Future projections: Non-clinical

Non-clinical situations are extremely varied. With a few exceptions, such as a major incident or black status due to a bed crisis or a labour ward being full, the majority of these situations will evolve over a longer time frame. They will not be perceived as immediately life threatening or being time critical, but they are more likely to fall into longer-term strategic planning. It will still be useful to use the mental rehearsal method of imagining different outcomes. This will feed into decision making which will be covered in Chapter 3.

Key points

- ◆ Situational awareness can be considered as comprising three components: perception, comprehension, and predicting future state.

- ◆ These three components echo the phrases 'what? so what? what next?'

- ◆ Perception for situational awareness at its most basic level involves a stimulus via sight, sound, or touch (occasionally, smell or taste).

◆ At a more complex level we also perceive self, risk, and time.

◆ We then make sense of what we have perceived and turn it into a mental model. This is our working idea of what we think we are dealing with.

◆ Barriers to perception and comprehension include high workload, time pressure, perceived high risk, stress, fatigue, biases (including expectation, confirmation, and environmental), task fixation, and inattentional blindness.

◆ Comprehension involves using a mixture of working memory and long-term memory. The latter involves recall of knowledge and past experience and may include pattern recognition of the cues.

◆ When building our mental model, problems can arise due to missed cues, misinterpreting cues, or choosing to ignore cues, incorrect risk assessment, poor time judgement, or a failure to update our mental model either when new information becomes available or when conditions change.

◆ To help with our mental model it is useful to commentate and share our thinking with our team. It is useful to compare the team's perceptions and understanding, and to incorporate these into a team mental model.

◆ The team needs a share understanding of the mental model.

◆ It can be useful to do a quick run-through of SHEEP to help with situational awareness. S—which guideline/SOP are we using? H—who is doing what? How is that working? E—are we in the best place to handle what we are managing? E—do we have all the kit that we need? P—how full is my bucket? Where is my focus? What are we doing about keeping time?

◆ It is useful to run through imaginary scenarios that project what may happen in the future to predict how things might progress.

◆ A different approach for future state planning may be needed in an emergency versus a routine of intermediate setting.

References

1. Endsley M. Toward a Theory of Situation Awareness in Dynamic Systems. *Human Factors* 1995; 37: 32–64.
2. Heifetz R. Leadership Without Easy Answers. Cambridge, MA: Belknap Press of Harvard University Press, 1994.
3. Miller G. The Magical Number Seven, Plus or Minus Two: Some Limits on our Capacity for Processing Information. *Psychological Review* 1956; 63: 81–97.
4. Weick KE. Puzzles in Organizational Learning: An Exercise in Disciplined Imagination. *British Journal of Management* 2002; 13: S7–15.

3

Decision making

I must have a prodigious quantity of mind; it takes me as much as a week, sometimes, to make it up.

Mark Twain, 1835–1910

The Innocents Abroad (1869)

Introduction

It is possible to consider decision making in two parts:[1–3]

1. the situational assessment (what's the problem?), and

2. the decision-making methods by which we come up with a plan of action (what shall I/we do?).

Situational assessment

There is an interface where comprehension of the current state (current mental model) that we alluded to as part of situational awareness starts to be explored in more depth. This is really the first step of decision making or the ***situational assessment***[2] (what's the problem here?).

I want to start to categorize broadly some of the ways that we might need to make decisions within healthcare settings. Like any attempt at classification it is a gross oversimplification but I want to try and unpick how we think in four different settings.

The four categories that I would like to consider are:

1 Acute/emergency

I want to include any process where there is a team of people under time pressure, emotional pressure, and which has a high cognitive workload. This is an unplanned or unexpected event. The team may start with just one individual and will expand as more help is called for when/if required.

In the past six months I have looked after a collapsed person in a super-market and another one outside a train station. I certainly wasn't expecting either of those events. It was a very different experience dealing with an emergency in an unfamiliar environment without the equipment or the people around that might be the 'norm'. I want to compare the emergency in an environment where you *are* expecting one versus the emergency in an environment where you *are not*.

2 Routine clinical

This category includes an enormous range of activities: ward work, outpatients, GP or dental surgery, routine lists of procedures, lab-based activities, pharmacy, and any other routine day-to-day experience. The routine 'stuff' covers everything that just ticks along when you are not being thrown the kinds of curve balls that fall into category 1.

The comprehension of situational awareness here will evolve into routine decision making and clinical reasoning. There are different barriers to doing this well than there are in an acute setting.

3 Routine becomes an emergency

This is a key type of situational-awareness issue that has caused error. The error occurs because we are 'stuck' in routine mode and don't pick up the cues that are flagging the fact that an emergency is developing.

We are particularly at risk if the emergency happens slowly over a longer time frame. Examples include the patient who has insufficient oral fluid intake for a number of days and gradually becomes dehydrated (perhaps right under our noses on a hospital ward); the slow bleed from a duodenal ulcer that happens overnight when observations are being taken less frequently and only in the morning is the drop in blood pressure detected (that is a very late sign); the decreased variability on a foetal trace that might indicate the baby isn't 'happy'; the gentle rise in carbon dioxide that initially goes unnoticed when malignant hyperthermia first presents itself but as it is so rare there is initial denial and the rise is attributed to others causes until it becomes barn door; the transient ischaemic attacks that are ignored as the symptoms resolve fairly quickly and the patient doesn't want to 'make a fuss'; the anaesthetic that should be routine in someone fit and healthy but has an unexpected difficult airway complication that goes unrecognized; the slow bleed during an operation where a bleeding blood vessel that is not in view is not noticed, or the gradual onset of sepsis in an inpatient admitted with another condition that goes undetected.

The early signs of an emergency may not be obvious. We must think about how we maintain our curiosity to keep looking for the unexpected. This skill involves how we keep on looking for today's gorilla (as in the film clip cited in Chapter 2) or how we improve our error awareness. There are both perceptive and comprehension elements involved. Only when we have the correct situational assessment of the emergency can we make the correct decisions about how to manage it.

4 **Non-clinical**

There are many people within healthcare working in entirely non-clinical roles. These may range from someone making decisions at a band 2 level to those making decisions at an executive or board level.

There are others who will perhaps gain more non-clinical decision-making responsibility as they progress through their clinical careers.

The decision making required in these settings is different from that required in a clinical setting. There will be a broad range of techniques employed.

An example of clinical decision making

At this point I want to introduce a real-life story. If you have time, grab a piece of paper and a pen. When I ask the questions try to scribble down a quick answer so that you are honest with yourself as the story progresses.

I want you to keep in mind the two steps of the process: the first part is defining what the condition might be, and the second part is deciding on the treatment.

It is possible for an error to occur with either:

1. the situational assessment (making the wrong diagnosis), and therefore choosing the wrong treatment (although it was the correct treatment for what you thought it was), or

2. the correct diagnosis is made and the wrong treatment is chosen, or the wrong course of action followed, or the treatment omitted.

See Example 3.1 and consider where the error occurred in this case and whether you would have made it too.

Example 3.1 True story

MF is a 45-year-old female who presents to her GP with indigestion pain. She is given gaviscon on a first visit and 'omeprazole equivalent' on her third presentation over about a two-month period.

What else would you like to know?

The other history that she offers up is that she is a smoker, she is treated for hypertension (not well controlled), and her husband died just over a year ago.

What would you do next as she sits in front of you? It is now her fourth visit?

As you are reading this example, I would imagine you are already guessing at the diagnosis. How are you doing that? I want you to think about how and what you are thinking (this is sometimes known as metacognition). Of course, the very fact that I am using the story alerts you to the fact that there was a problem and is altering the way that you are thinking.

Why is it different to pull together cues as I list them for you from the more complex process if you were taking the history yourself? If you are sitting in a clinic and this is the fourth visit from this patient and it is the tenth patient today and you are running 20 minutes late, how might your thought processes be affected by these external factors?

Let us return to the story. During the fourth visit, MF suggests that her indigestion is still not controlled and that it is interfering with her exercise regime, which is important to her as she is trying to lose some weight.

What questions might you wish to ask to inform your situational assessment?

Had the questions been asked you would know that the pain sometimes radiates into her jaw and down her arms. Oh, and there is a family history of coronary heart disease.

However, these questions were not asked and so the information remained hidden from the GP and a referral for a routine endoscopy was organized.

On the night of our main story, MF has the worst indigestion she has ever had. She has consumed 'gallons' of gaviscon with no relief. It is night-time but she can't sleep, 'if I could just get rid of this pain!' After hours of severe pain, she finally calls an ambulance. The paramedics are initially rather dismissive asking why she hasn't called her GP first. She has no relief from the first 'shot' of morphine and the second dose doesn't touch the pain either, although she is now as 'high as a kite and spacey'. The paramedics listen to the story: 'if I could just chop my jaw off and my arms off, I feel like the pain would go away'.

They perform an ECG and state that it is not her heart, but in view of the fact that the morphine hasn't worked that maybe they should take her in, just in case.

What are your thoughts? How are you making decisions? How would you clarify or confirm your thoughts?

On arrival in the emergency department further history is taken ('I'm under investigation for indigestion, I wonder if I might have an ulcer?'), some baseline observations reveal a very high blood pressure. A repeat ECG is met with a confirmation: 'it's not your heart! We will organize an urgent endoscopy. I'm not sure what time it will be. I'll just go and get that organized.'

What are your thoughts now? How did you reach that decision? What would you do next?

Her 16-year-old daughter, J, accompanies MF into the emergency department.

'I feel a bit faint, I think I might pass out', says MF to J. J stands and walks around the trolley to pour out a glass of water. As J returns to the bedside, her mother collapses and appears to be shaking. J calls for help. Two people come into the cubicle but then leave again. J runs to the reception desk and grabs the phone out of someone's hand and drags her to help her mother whom she thinks is being ignored. The other two people return (we assume that one collected the crash trolley and the other pulled an emergency bell). A full crash team arrives. After two shocks circulation is restored. J has just witnessed her mum being resuscitated, aged 16, after losing her dad only just over a year ago.

M is rushed to the cardiology unit. Three stents are inserted. (The endoscopy is cancelled.) Widespread narrowing of the arterial supply to the heart is discovered, as is a high cholesterol level. Treatment is commenced for her heart, her cholesterol, and her blood pressure.

What are your thoughts and feelings now?

Of course, there are lots of positives. A life has been saved. Thank goodness she was in the emergency department and not at home. A great big thank-you is due to the team that got her back.

However, my thoughts and feelings are mixed.

Could this all have been prevented if it was picked up earlier?

And the 16-year-old daughter who only lost her father a year ago? What are your thoughts and feelings about her?

How can we learn from this episode?

MF is my friend and she is keen that we learn from this. She gave me permission to tell you her story. She doesn't want to blame anyone, but she would like to know that we can learn from her story and use this to improve what we do.

I want you to think hard about cues, pattern recognition, intuition, experience, and gut instinct.

If I say to you 'central chest pain' and you are a clinician, I can probably influence the way you are thinking by adding in 'trigger words'. If I say 'crushing' or 'like an elephant sitting on your chest', I can probably nudge your thoughts towards a cardiac cause. I can do this even more so if I add 'radiates to jaw or left arm'. What if I add in 'sweaty and clammy'?

We start again and now I say, 'chest pain that is mild and relieved by gaviscon. It is worse with spicy food or when the patient leans forwards.' What are you thinking now? Have I moved your thoughts towards a gastro-intestinal cause?

We start again: now I tell you that she is experiencing chest pain that radiates to the back. Now what are you thinking?

Now I want you to think about *how* you are thinking.

I am presenting you a few words written on a page. You are potentially seeing those words (perceiving) and choosing them from within the sentence (filtering) and linking them with other chosen words (pattern formation). This involves a sort of matching process in our memory banks. We build a pattern in front of us and match it to something we have seen before or learnt about before. We are searching for an answer or solution to **'what's the problem?'**

What is it about either the way we are trained or what we have experienced that leads us towards this pattern recognition of cues? Is it a good idea? My answer is both yes and no. Of course, if we are to make a diagnosis we need to construct the correct mental model and build towards a working diagnosis. However, if we jump to the mental model too early we run the risk of introducing bias. We may sift through the information and simply filter out the bits that don't fit with what we have already decided the mental model should be. How can we make sure that we don't filter too early in the story or jump to an early conclusion and then fail to ask the right questions or gather the right information?

When I was a house officer (newly qualified doctor), I was encouraged to state what my diagnosis (symbol Δ) was at the very end of every admission. (An admission involved taking a history, performing an examination, taking observations and documenting them.) To follow my diagnosis, I was always encouraged to write a list of differentials (symbol $\Delta\Delta$). This list of differential diagnoses or 'what else could it be?' was something I didn't really grasp the importance of at the time. I am not sure if I'm having a nostalgic, rose-tinted moment when I think back and reflect that more emphasis was placed on this when I was younger than is with house-officer equivalents (currently called F1s) today. I think there was almost a competitive element to see who could come up with the longest list of differentials (but perhaps that was just me). I was, however, reassured at a recent conference by a medical student that enormous emphasis is being placed on this in current training.

Following the list of differentials we documented a list of investigations that would be required to help us explore which of our possible diagnoses might be the correct one. (I am not sure this process has changed much over the past 20 years other than perhaps there are now fancier tests, and the Internet is available to use as a cognitive resource.)

We will return to the idea of when it is appropriate to try to weigh up all the different options before we make a diagnosis and when in other settings it might be necessary to act first and ask more questions later. Two important factors are the time pressure or urgency and the perceived seriousness/risk of the situation.

The reason that we don't want to lose sight of this 'differential' concept is that it stops us getting stuck in the 'assumption' that the first mental model we choose is the correct one. It encourages us to think broadly—what else could it be? Why isn't it one of these other things? How can I make sure I'm not missing something here?

As more information is uncovered (blood results are back, X-ray now taken, information from the previous admission is now available, a relative arrives who told us something else that was relevant, we have managed to speak to the person's GP to fill in some gaps), we may wish to change our working diagnosis and, at the very least, we should review it in light of the new information.

I want us to concentrate hard on this concept of thinking of a diagnosis as not something that is set in stone, but instead something that is reviewed and reconsidered throughout our clinician--patient interaction. We cannot treat something successfully if we don't know what it is!

I hope you will remember my two friends (Mrs D and MF, see Level One, p. 14) time and time again if you ever need reminding about why this is important.

Whilst we have referred to the term DODAR for decision making in Level One (which like many things in the field of human factors came from the aviation industry),[1,4] I want to introduce a different mnemonic here: DECIDE (also originally from aviation), which I've adapted for use in healthcare (see Figure 3.1 and Figure 3.2).

I have started with a fairly simple system, a sort of big-picture approach to decision making. This mnemonic has been developed in two versions for clinical and non-clinical decision making (Figures 3.1 and Figure 3.2 respectively).

After considering this broad-based system, we will explore things in more depth.

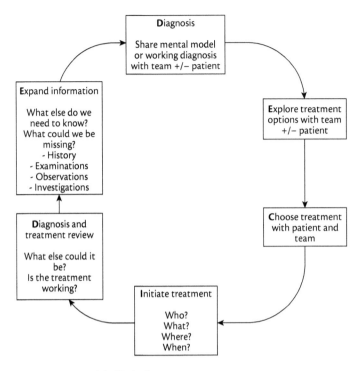

Figure 3.1 DECIDE model: Clinical.

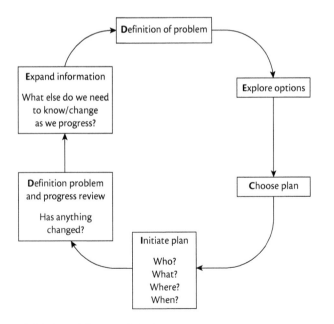

Figure 3.2 DECIDE model: Non-clinical.

DECIDE for a clinical diagnosis

I want to emphasize that the processes within the DECIDE model are displayed as a circle for a reason; it encourages ongoing diagnostic review.

The clinical version starts by sharing the working *diagnosis* (D) or mental model with the team by verbalizing it.

Once the diagnosis is made, the team *explores* (E) the treatment options.

The team then *chooses* (C) one or more of these treatment options.

It may sound daft, but the next step is actually to make sure the treatment is *initiated* (I). There are multiple times in simulation where I have witnessed the team thoroughly exploring the option-generation phase but they then fail to initiate the treatment. This involves thinking about *who* is doing *what* by *when*.

The next step is to review the *diagnosis* (D) and the progress of the condition with the current treatment. This can be considered in three steps.

◆ What else could this be?

◆ What is happening with the progress of the baseline disease?

◆ What effect is the treatment having?

The final step before we continue the next cycle involves *expanding* (E) on the information that is available.

◆ What are we missing here?

◆ Do we need any further history?

◆ Review the history.

◆ Repeat examination.

◆ Repeat observations.

◆ What other investigations might be useful?

◆ Review all the results and chase any missing results.

Then go back to the beginning and repeat DECIDE.

DECIDE for a non-clinical problem

This model is also envisaged as a circle in order to encourage regular review of both the problem and progress made.

The *definition* (D) of the problem is shared with the team.

The team *explores* (E) management options or solutions.

The team *chooses* (C) a solution or plan.

The solution or plan is *initiated* (I), with clear allocation of who is doing what by when.

Both the *definition* (D) of the problem and the solution are reviewed as the plan progresses.

As the plan progresses it may be useful to *expand* (E) the information available. What else might we need to know? Who else might need to be informed or involved? Do all our stakeholders know what we are trying to achieve here?

When we start again with the next cycle, it is worth considering whether we had a full grasp of what the problem really is.

DECIDE in practice

Using Figure 3.1 I want you to consider another real example. Example 3.2 is again about somebody I know, this time a male relative who has volunteered his story so that we may learn from it. I am also trying to include some more primary-care examples in this book so that we do not think that human factors study has to focus solely on hospitals (this has been requested by a couple of my GP colleagues).

Example 3.2 Another real story

Please have a look at Figure 3.1 before you start.

TL is a fit and healthy 40-year-old male. He is a non-smoker, eats healthily, takes a moderate amount of exercise, and has no significant past medical history nor family history.

On this day, he presents to his GP with a pain in his lower leg. He has never had anything like this before.

If we try to take assumptions away and just think about a leg. What is in a leg?

In the most basic terms it is muscle, bone, fat, tendons, blood vessels, skin, and a bit of connective tissue. Can you think of something that could be wrong with each of those in a leg, please? If you have time, try to scribble them on a piece of paper but please stop for a moment and give this some thought. We should have a list of at least five things that might be wrong with a leg.

Now, as we examine the leg, we can be pondering those five things and asking ourselves 'is there anything else it could be?'

I suspect that this was not the order of thought processes in this particular doctor's mind. Of course, I am making an assumption, but TL reports that the doctor quickly examined the leg, established that the calf was rather tender, and suggested some pain killers for the 'strained muscle'.

From what was on your list of five, would anything else fit with a tender calf muscle?

TL gave himself a firm talking to and went to work the next day despite a leg that felt worse. As the day progressed, he seemed to be developing another pain. This time it was in his chest. Perhaps he was a bit run down or he was coming down with something?

The pain was in the back of his chest on the right. I want you to think about what structures are there. From the outside in we find skin, subcutaneous tissues and fat, bone, intercostal muscles, neurovascular bundles, pleura, potential space between the pleura, lung (airways and blood vessels), referred pain from somewhere else (diaphragm, heart, gastro-intestinal). Now think of something that could cause pain involving as many of those as possible.

Now consider both those that link with a pain in the leg and those that don't. They could be connected but they could also be separate.

TL returned to his GP the next day to report the worsening condition of his leg and his new added symptom of pain in his chest.

If you were this GP, with your list of conditions that might be related and might not be, what would you be paying attention to on your examination? What investigations might you need to perform?

Would you send him home, observe him, or send him into hospital? How would you make that decision?

Are you using pattern recognition or gut instinct? Have you done sufficient option generation? How confident are you in your decision? What caveats might you consider to back up your choice of diagnosis? How would you make sure that your decision is reviewed?

TL had some blood tests but was sent home and went back to work. He became increasingly short of breath and on returning home that night, his wife took him to hospital.

The diagnosis was a deep vein thrombosis (DVT) and pulmonary embolus (PE). By this time he was severely hypoxic (very low oxygen levels) and the diagnosis was now quite clear with the passage of time and his deterioration.

How did you do?

If you reached the correct conclusion, that's great, especially as you were unable to actually see the patient or examine him. But I would still like you to think about how you reached it.

If, like the GP, you didn't manage to put the pieces together, can you retrace your thought processes and keep an eye open for any assumptions you might have made along the way?

The GP concerned was experienced (GP for over 30 years) and well respected. We can all make mistakes. How are you going to change your practice to reduce your chance of making the next one?

In both of the cases above (TL and MF) the error came at the situational-assessment phase of decision making; that is, problem definition.

If the diagnosis had indeed been a gastric problem, then endoscopy would be an appropriate course of action. If the second diagnosis was a simple muscle strain, then some analgesia would be appropriate.

The DECIDE model rather oversimplifies matters. When we start to dig into things in a bit more depth there is a lot more complexity involved.

Acute/emergency setting

I want us to introduce a pattern of thinking for this setting to try to help with the situational assessment and also to feed into the situational awareness of the projection to the future state. We need to ensure that we have used our current awareness of the situation to feed into our decision-making process.

I am going to take you back to Endlsey's 'what, so what, what next?' triad,[5] but then adapt it by throwing in a bit of SHEEP.

1. *What* are we dealing with here?

   Verbalize the working diagnosis to the rest of the team (sharing the mental model for the current state).

   Consider also: 'What am I missing here? What else could this be?'

2. Now do the SHEEP version of *so what*? (SHEEP awareness)

   ◆ S—which guideline/plan are we using for this? What other treatment options/management plans could we consider? Do we need any more cognitive aids?

◆ H—have we got the right people in the room and have they all been allocated tasks appropriately? Are they performing those tasks competently? Do we have a time keeper if appropriate or a timescale in which we need to solve this?

◆ E—are we in the right place for this situation; if so, is it optimized for what we are dealing with? If not, where should we be and how do we get there?

◆ E—have we got the right kit here and people who know how to use it?

◆ P—how full is my bucket? Do I need help?

3. **What next**? (Repeat SHEEP for future projection.)

◆ S—what other guidelines might be relevant as this episode progresses? Where are the guidelines? Can we access them either electronically or in paper form and bring them to the bedside?

◆ H—who else will we need? Will we need different expertise or simply more people? Where are they now and how long will it take them to get here?

◆ E—do we need to be moving somewhere else? How are we going to get there? (Links with H—who do we need to make that move? Links with E—what equipment will we need for that move?)

◆ E—what other kit will we need? Where is the kit? How are we going to get it ready?

◆ P—how full will my bucket become if this unravels? What else might I need to be aware of?

I want to explore the '***what***?' *What* are we dealing with here? *What* is the problem? *What* is the diagnosis? *What* is the shared mental model?

The next thing that I want to explore is how do we decide *what* the '*what*' is?

The first thing I think we need to decide is whether we are dealing with an emergency or not—in other words, do we need to act quickly because this is either high risk or time critical?

I want you to try to visualize each of the patients I am about to describe. I want you to ask yourself in each case, is this an emergency or not? This is the most superficial situational assessment that we need to make.

◆ Patient unexpectedly found unconscious in his bed. Emergency or not?

◆ Patient in the waiting room of an orthopaedic clinic complaining of crushing central chest pain and looking cyanosed. Emergency or not?

♦ You are in a supermarket and turn a corner to see someone fitting on the floor. Emergency or not?

♦ As you enter a labour ward-room you are met with a sight of the blood pressure machine reading 80/50 and a large pool of blood on the floor. Emergency or not?

♦ A baby is brought in to you who hasn't been feeding well, has had diarrhoea, and is now floppy and unresponsive. Emergency or not?

♦ Following a dental abscess, the swelling in the patient's neck means that they are having difficulty swallowing their own saliva. Emergency or not?

♦ Sudden loss of power in both legs and faecal incontinence. Emergency or not?

♦ Asthma attack severe enough that there is a silent chest and the person is unable to talk in sentences. Emergency or not?

♦ Anaesthetist can't intubate, has lost control of the airway, and the saturations are dropping. Emergency or not?

♦ The laboratory processing the results for my patient shuts in 30 minutes and it is Friday on a bank holiday weekend. I need this result to plan my patient's care for the next three days. Emergency or not?

♦ There is a person standing on the bridge threatening to jump. Emergency or not?

If you have worked in a patient-facing role for any length of time, I bet you are thinking, 'too easy!'

Why is that?

I have given you different ages of patients in different specialties and in different environments. How have you established the facts in such a short space of time?

How are you making your initial assessment? How long did you think about it for? Why is that?

In an emergency setting we need to act quickly. A number of the examples above are extremely time critical (minutes) whilst others are urgent but you might have slightly longer to start a definitive treatment or to take action before things become critical.

Thus we are taking cues that we have perceived and assessing whether we think they are high risk and how long we might have to sort the problem out.

This is stage one of the decision-making process—i.e. emergency or not? We may or may not be able to define the problem at this stage but we can act anyway.

If we establish that it is an emergency, we may simply initiate action as per our previous experience or by invoking a guideline. If it is not an urgent setting then we have more time to explore our situation assessment in much more detail.

Let's start to explore what the next stage of decision making might entail.

Decision-making possibilities for selecting a treatment or action

Using a naturalistic approach, it has been suggested that there are four main ways that decisions are made.[1-3,5,6]

1. Option generation and choice

2. Rule-based

3. Intuitive or recognition-primed

4. Creative

My thoughts are that this approach infers that there are four *distinct* ways of making decisions. In reality I think the boundaries between them are often blurred. I also believe that we don't always complete the situation assessment prior to initiating the treatment. I think the initial treatment may be started as a holding measure while we gather more information. I also recognize that we might employ some of these techniques whilst still at the problem-definition phase. As I have already suggested, option generation around diagnosis—that is, generating a list of differentials—can help us to keep our options open and to reduce the chance of cognitive bias as new information is gathered.

However, I think it is useful to explore what these categories of decision making entail and to illustrate this with real examples.

Option generation and choice

We have already begun to explore option generation. We might generate options about what the problem might be and then choose one. We might then generate options regarding possible courses of action or treatments and then choose which of those fits our situation best.

One option may be to do nothing, something often known as expectant management. It was described to me when I was a junior as 'masterly inactivity and cat-like observation'. Following the principle of 'first, do no harm', it can be best not to jump straight in and act. It can be more difficult to pause instead, and to watch like mad.

I have witnessed this occurring many times in theatre with the experienced versus the novice surgeon. The more senior surgeon more readily waits to let a clot form on a bleeding piece of tissue rather than keep on dabbing at it and repeatedly disturbing the clot. It is harder to stand there and appear to be doing nothing when you perceive a whole theatre is watching and waiting for you to solve the problem. Waiting and taking time to observe comes with confidence and experience, and I have seen how useful it can be with tonsillectomies, caesarean sections, or an open prostatectomy, dental extraction, or a laparotomy.

After a patient is admitted it may be that the diagnosis is not yet clear. For example, perhaps there are some features of a possible appendicitis but it is certainly not a barn door diagnosis. A conservative approach in this setting may avoid unnecessary surgery.

It is always worth considering the options of doing nothing or doing nothing yet.

We generally need time to use this method of generating options, although how long it takes will depend on how often we have faced a similar setting. If we face the condition regularly then the options may generate themselves almost automatically. A word of caution when you find yourself in this familiar setting; the automated response can have built-in complacency.

I ask you to remain curious, to double-check with yourself, every time you are presented with a setting you are very familiar with and especially those which seem either mundane or trivial. Have I got the diagnosis right? Am I missing anything here? Is there anything else we should have considered or done?

Always expect the unexpected (this is sometimes known as the 'black-swan' approach).

Aside: The black swan[7]

How do you know to look for something if you don't know it exists? Pre-eighteenth century, no-one had ever seen a black swan. An assumption was made that all swans are white. I want you to look for black swans (or the gorillas or moon-walking bears I mentioned in Chapter 1). *In other words, I want you to remain alert and curious and wonder what today's error might be. Then you can plan how to prevent it happening. If you aren't looking for it, how will you stop it?*

In a setting where we have more time available we can discuss everything with our team and gather all of their thoughts. We can spend time weighing up the advantages, risks, and disadvantages of each particular option that is put forward. We can consult with experts (locally or regionally or beyond), textbooks, papers, the British National Formulary, and any other relevant resources. We can hold multi-professional meetings to gather opposing views in order to make the final treatment decision more informed. Once we have implemented this chosen treatment option, we then review that decision and the progress of the treatment, trying to dissect the underlying course of the disease from the impact of the treatment.

Remember also that when we use option generation to make our list of differential diagnosis and choose one for our working diagnosis this decision also needs reviewing. Have we got the diagnosis right? Is there any new information that has shifted the goalposts?

In an emergency setting we may initiate cardiac massage and follow resuscitation guidelines. Once supportive measures are underway we may then get to option generation, known as the 4Hs and 4Ts (hypoxia, hypovolaemia, hypothermia, hyper/hypokalaemia or metabolic, and thrombolic, tension pneumothorax, tamponade, and toxic/therapeutic). Here is a rule and a mnemonic that have been developed to help as *aides memoire* to use when we are stressed, when we have a 'full bucket'. It is very difficult to develop a quick check list of how to go about something in an emergency setting, so this is done for us. Once tried and tested, this method was then introduced as standard: a rule-based approach for option generation and taught nationally on resuscitation courses.

We can use the mnemonic as a pre-taught, shared mental model to help us decide which of these options may have led to the cardiac arrest and therefore what treatment we might need to consider which will correct it. So that even in this time-pressured setting we can be sure that we are still covering all of the options.

This leads us to the next type of decision making: rule-based decision making.

Rule-based

When we identify a cardiac arrest we start using a guideline/protocol. This is produced as an algorithm which displays a flow diagram with a series of actions that we should follow. In theory at least, everyone who is part of a cardiac arrest team, whilst they may never have met each other before, should have been trained in a standardized way to deal with this particular emergency.

They should know that they need a leader, clear team roles, a time keeper, and the lists of actions that they should all be following.

By having a shared mental model of how to manage a cardiac arrest and by following the rules that are in place, the decision making that is required during that stressful setting should be markedly reduced. We know how long the cycles are, which drugs we are giving when, when, and if to deliver a shock, how to go about that, and we have rules for managing the airway. This allows our cognitive ability to be focused on how to problem solve what the underlying issue might be using the 4Hs and 4Ts.

Having a clear protocol or guideline that we can use in any emergency setting makes a lot of sense. We know that our stress hormones will be coming into play and that our bucket will be relatively full at this time. The majority of guidelines for emergencies are written in the cold light of day when the experts producing the guideline are not coping with a full bucket.

Back to our setting. Of course, we have to realize it is an emergency. Whilst saying, 'this is an emergency' and starting a holding measure of ABCDE (airway, breathing, circulation, dysfunction, and everything else) (a rule-based approach) may stand us in good stead for a time, it will not solve every emergency.

Once we have realized what we are seeing *is* an emergency, it is helpful to know which one we are witnessing. We have to recognize it. This brings us to the next type of decision making: recognition-primed or intuitive.

Intuitive or recognition-primed

This is the method where we somehow inherently know what we should be doing—we go with our 'gut instinct'. That doesn't sound terribly scientific, does it?

What we are actually doing is very fast, almost automatic, pattern recognition. In some cases it may be so fast that we are practically missing out the situational-assessment phase and leaping straight into an action. You could argue that recognizing a cardiac arrest and starting CPR falls into this category; we act before we start to think about the rules that we are following.

(I am going to use anaesthetic examples in this section as of course my recognition-primed responses will naturally occur in my background specialty.)

The first step is to pick up on the cues, the risks, the time factor, and speed of action required. How quickly we identify the cues (salient points of the history, examination, observations, and investigations) and pull the pieces together to make something recognizable depends on many things including: our past experience, knowledge, stress levels, fatigue, memory recall, pattern recognition, time pressure, level of expertise, how obvious it is that there is a problem (car crash, unconscious person lying in a large pool of blood), any other distractions that we are facing simultaneously, and which emergency we most recently saw or read about or heard about at a meeting.

An expert will have more experience on which to base a 'gut instinct' than the novice, who may have to resort to first principles and try to problem solve from scratch.

This intuitive method links with the 'thinking fast and slow' model proposed by Professor Kahneman.[8] His theory proposed that humans have two systems for decision making; a fast, automatic mode (system 1), and a second slow, deliberate, and rational mode (system 2). Whilst we like to think of ourselves as logical beings who weigh up options and really think things through, he discovered that we are over-reliant on the fast system. We make potentially between 2000 and 10 000 decisions per day and so most of them need to happen quickly and without conscious effort. System 1 happens effortlessly and is responsible for most of what we do. If you look up now, what can you see? It is system 1 that tells you that is a wall or a door or a tree, your visual perception.

If I ask you 'what is 2 + 2', the answer 4 will just appear using system 1. If however, I now ask you to calculate your body-mass index correct to one decimal place, the much slower and deliberate system 2 would be called upon (see Example 3.3).

Example 3.3 Testing system 2

Using system 2 fills up your bucket. It generates a high cognitive workload. If you would like to test this for yourself here are a couple of things to try. I want you to start with the classic 'pat your head and rub your tummy'. So with one hand you gently and regularly pat your head whilst the other hand makes a circular action rubbing your tummy. Now start to recite the alphabet backwards.

How far did you get? If you got stuck, did you automatically stop moving your hands to allow yourself to think?

If you get up from where you are and go for a walk and at the same time repeatedly double the number starting with the number 2 (i.e. 2, 4, 8, 16, and so on), how far did you get? Did you have to stop walking first to get to that number?

Whilst we may consider our decision making to be better represented by our system 2, the truth is actually that system 1 seems to be much more powerful. The two systems can end up in opposition and the result can be a cognitive bias. This bias can result in a predictable systematic error.

For example, the outcome of the most recent case we saw with a particular condition can influence our decision the next time we see that condition. This is known as the 'anchoring effect'. Fast system 1 takes over and says, 'I've seen this before, I know the answer to this problem'. The fast system takes a short cut and bypasses logic. This is how it causes a bias.

Another example. An underlying subconscious thought process might be as follows: 'I'm in day-case theatre. This is where we do routine operations. This is not where emergencies happen.' These are examples of environmental or perhaps expectation biases.

The 'halo effect' and the 'hero effect': the former is when we like something so we assume that everything to do with it is positive, and the latter is the person equivalent; we like someone, so we assume that all of his or her decisions are correct. The converse is true in that if we don't' like something, we may assume that everything to do with it is negative.

These biases are important to recognize and as yet not enough attention has been given to the systems and equipment we use, and the environment we work in, to help 'design out' these bias traps that we fall into.

So, bearing in mind that our intuition can take us the wrong way, let us continue to explore some of those intuitive or recognition-primed responses. As we explore these I want you to stay curious: ask yourself, could there be a down side to the assumptions we are making when trusting gut instinct?

There are different degrees of recognition-primed (RP) responses.[1,2,6]

Simple recognition-primed

In anaesthetics there are lots of tips that we acquire by means of the apprenticeship style of our training. We work with senior colleagues who have developed wonderful gems to pass on.

The following were all shared with me when I was a trainee, in a non-acute setting. To set the context, they are between 10 and 20 years old.

> 'Try a half twist as you insert the LMA (laryngeal mask airway) for this one.'

> 'Rotate it anticlockwise as you insert it (the tracheal tube on a bougie).'

> 'Use lignocaine gel on the nasopharyngeal airway, it's better tolerated.'

> 'Just move the head like this ... there you go, it goes in more easily like that (blind nasal intubation).'

> 'As they are waking up, they yawn, it's a perfect time to take it out (paediatric LMA).'

> 'When there is a leak like that around the LMA in an edentulous patient, try inserting two rolled gauze swabs that is prepared as a sausage like this.'

Each of these is not a rule that is written down anywhere. Each top tip or solution to a problem was something that might have originally fallen into the creative decision-making category but was then passed from one generation of anaesthetists to the next.

It becomes a link: thoughts of 'see this pattern, perform this action' or 'I have seen this before, we tried that and it worked, I'll try that again' may well be going through our brains but the thoughts may be at a subconscious level. The action becomes automatic.

More complex recognition-primed

Let us increase the urgency of the situation and think about an episode of brady-cardia (slow heart rate) in a patient during an operation. In certain types of surgery (those with a chance of evoking a vagal response, for example, eye surgery, laparoscopy, anal stretch, some gynaecological surgery) we might be expecting that this response is more likely to occur. We will have anticipated the need to give a drug to bring the heart rate up again. Those who are risk averse (I put myself in this group) would already have the correct drug drawn up and ready to administer. Different anaesthetists will have a preference for different drugs in this setting but any option generation will largely have taken place in advance. When the pattern recognition occurs—a change in rate of the beeps (auditory cue), change in the ECG waveform, the numeric reading, and pulse oximeter waveform (visual including waveform patterns and numerical data), with perhaps a change in blood pressure or even end tidal CO_2 waveform with or without an alarm sounding (more auditory), possibly the anaesthetist will take the pulse (touch)—the experienced anaesthetist will have set a threshold at which he or she will act.

Whilst there is a rule-based approach to this scenario, I would hazard a guess that if we had a room full of experienced anaesthetists we would find each took a slightly different approach, tailor-made to the specific situation at hand. They may all say that their approach is based on experience but in fact it would fall into the category of a recognition-primed response.

Added complexity: Recognition-primed

Let us imagine another level of complexity. There is a sudden, significant, unexpected drop in blood pressure during the operation. Assuming we have confirmed that it is not an erroneous reading but is indeed a genuine drop in blood pressure, we will rapidly have decided what we think it might be. In broad terms the patient may be underfilled (blood loss or fluid loss or fluid in the wrong space), the patient could be vasodilated (blood vessels opened up), or there could be a pump problem (heart not pumping as well as it should be).

If an experienced anaesthetist was managing the case he or she will 'have a feel' of where the patient is with regards to filling, level of vasodilation, and whether the 'pump' is an issue. This anaesthetist will almost simultaneously be able to decide which of the solutions should be tried first, and what order the other options should be tried if the first doesn't work.

An aside

If you were to push me hard and say that 'a feel' doesn't sound terribly comforting or evidenced based, and ask me 'where does the 'feel' come from?' then I would have to give you a long list of contributory factors that would all help to build up the picture that results in this instinct: pre-operative—the history, the examination, and the observations, past anaesthetics, notes, pre-operative fluid balance, things you might notice when you put the cannula in, ease with which you find a vein, speed of induction, how much anaesthetic required, haemodynamic stability on induction, rate and rhythm, swing on the pleth trace, urine output, blood loss, other losses, how much fluid the patient already needed and how he or she responded to filling, and so on. There is no formula to tell you what weight to place on each of those factors; you learn to juggle all of the cues and build an overall 'gut feeling' of what they represent.

Back to the patient.

Once a treatment choice is initiated, staff will more actively search for the reason it has failed and see how this matches the initial option chosen. (A word of caution about confirmation bias at this point. Remember that even when we are experienced, we tend to pick up or pay attention to those cues that fit with what we think the problem is.)

Staff may well run through some mental rehearsals of how things might progress, how they would handle specific scenarios should they occur, and what they might need. Hopefully they would share the mental model and possible future projections with the team, and then prepare anything else that might be required.

I have heard a lot in my years in anaesthetics of the difference between the science and the art of anaesthesia. I find myself wondering if the 'art' bit is the recognition-primed anaesthesia? However, we also need to know when there may be a bias sneaking up on us from that fast system 1.

Creative

In an emergency, there is rarely time for a creative response. This type of decision making is usually seen in a non-acute setting when we are facing a problem that we have never seen before or about which we have no knowledge. It can also be true when we are innovating and trying a novel solution to a known problem.

There is a well-known story of a surgeon and his colleague being on an aeroplane when someone developed a tension pneumothorax (collapsed lung with air around the outside of it). As they had no equipment available they managed to use what was available (including a coat hanger and a plastic bottle) to construct a life-saving chest drain equivalent. This would be an example of a creative solution being found despite the emergency pressure of the situation and lack of familiarity with the environment, and lack of availability of the usual equipment and staff.

As it happens, I have my own personal story that would also fit this bill (see Example 3.4).

Example 3.4 Henry the Hoover and Humphrey the Straw

Over eight years ago, my dad was coming towards the end of his battle with cancer. During the last week or so of his life, we were brilliantly supported by the local Macmillan unit who visited at least daily. This enabled us to keep him at home for his dying days as he had wanted.

My sisters and I took turns at night to sit by his side. On one particular night, I noticed at 2 a.m. that his secretions were suddenly becoming a real issue. He was unconscious and no longer swallowing but I was determined that he was not going to choke! Wiping them away seemed to resemble a little boy on a man's errand; of course what we really needed was a suction unit.

My weary brain decided that the answer must lie with Henry the Hoover (other brands would have performed just as well). The next thing I needed to replicate was a Yankauer sucker with a hole in it. What on earth did we have at home that could possibly fit the bill? I called one of my sisters in to be with Dad and went off to rummage in the kitchen, looking for something tube-like with a bend in it that would be acceptable to put into someone's mouth. I opened kitchen cupboards at random, scanning each shelf. And then it came to me, what I needed was a drinking straw.

When I was growing up, there was an advertisement made by the Milk Marketing Board. There was a straw called Humphrey and the idea was that you should drink your milk quickly or Humphrey might sneak up around a corner and steal it from you. The slogan was 'watch out, watch out, there's a Humphrey about', or at least that is how I remember it. I suddenly found myself chanting the slogan!

The drinking straw was fit for purpose. It normally goes into one's mouth, it had a flexible bit for easy adjustment, and it was soft enough to cut easily. I started cutting a hole small enough to fit my finger over so that I could regulate the strength of the suction. Perfect; a home-made Yankauer!

Now I needed something to go between the end of the Hoover and the straw. I managed to use a freezer bag and some sticky tape. At this point I had a slightly surreal, 'Blue Peter' moment. I taped the end of the straw inside a small hole that I had made in the freezer bag. I then taped the contraption onto the long hose of the Hoover. I performed a quick test with some water from a cup. Success! I think by now both my mum and my sleeping sister were both awake and wondering why I had decided to vacuum the house at such an ungodly hour.

I then performed a team-training session on how to suction safely. (None of the rest of my family members is medically trained. I suspect it was perhaps one of my least well-planned sessions but I think I made up for it with enthusiasm and relief and a bit of 3 a.m. mania.) I sound a bit flippant considering the seriousness of the situation but we had to keep our sense of humour to stop us giving up and sobbing in a crumpled heap. My dad was known for always being a joker and we were teasing him constantly as we cared for him.

Relieved that we were now able to keep him comfortable, we returned to bed.

After a couple of days, a suction unit was found for us to have at home and my Heath Robinson construction could go to rest.

Of course, I could have made my decisions differently rather than take the creative route that seemed to emerge naturally. I could have 'option-generated' ideas about who might have a suction unit or called an ambulance. It is difficult to know why I didn't call anyone. Did I was worry that my 2 a.m. mental model of an 'ambulance' might want to take him to hospital and I knew that wasn't what he wanted? Was I trying not to disturb fellow health professionals in the middle of the night? Who knows? I was horribly sleep deprived and my bucket was certainly very full.

Creative decision making is more commonly seen in a situation that is low risk and without time pressure. We will consider it further in those settings.

Routine clinical

Imagine now that we have removed the risk of the emergency situation. Even if this is the case, in healthcare other time pressures are incredibly common. Think of time pressure related to the workload of an overbooked clinic, a 6-minute time slot for a consultation, or an understaffed ward.

Let us move towards a nirvana of decision making when we have enough time to explore both the diagnostic decisions and the treatment decisions in a routine setting.

One of the key things that will influence whether we get the diagnosis correct is the information we gather. This information will take many forms: the auditory route as the patient (plus or minus relatives) shares his or her history, written information (notes—which may be vast and need serious weeding through to get to the essence of what we need to know, referral letters) which add to the patient's story, sight and touch as we observe and examine findings, and further data in various forms as we gather observations (height, weight, blood pressure, heart rate, saturations) and investigation results (urine dipstick, blood glucose, blood results, X-rays, ECG, or other more specialist data).

We have talked already about gathering this information to build into a mental model and how we then do this in more detail as our situational assessment. What is this?

We have already discussed how what you are expecting to see (that day, in that clinic/ward, with that patient) will influence what you see. This is the expectation bias. There is also confirmation bias to consider—perhaps the diagnosis has been made by someone else, perhaps you made the diagnosis yourself on a previous visit, and we do not routinely challenge this diagnosis or review it.

The three most likely decision-making methods that are used in this setting are option-generation, rule-based, and sometimes creative methods. We should not have to rely on our gut instinct or recognition-primed approach. Whilst these may give us a 'hunch' about which diagnosis may be favoured or what the best treatment might be, we should be able to take enough time to weigh things up and broaden our options to make sure we have not waded in and fallen into the bias traps mentioned above. Of course, with experience the choices may be considered quite rapidly, but do try to remain curious and think about the black swan that may suddenly swim up alongside you and present you with the entirely unexpected, even it is just a fleeting thought.

Option generation

Option generation is common in this setting. We produce a list of differential diagnoses as already discussed and opt for a working diagnosis. The treatment options are (hopefully) discussed clearly with the patient and his or her input influences the choice where possible. See the DECIDE mode (Figures 3.1 and 3.2).

Rule-based

It may be that there is a protocol or guideline that exists. In this case the first step is to make the diagnosis and match it to the protocol/guideline. This is more complicated than it sounds.

It involves gathering of the correct information, processing it, putting the cues together into a pattern that is recognizable (situation assessment or problem definition—what is it?), and then recognizing that a guideline/protocol exists for that problem. Either the protocol must be learnt or recalled (accurately?), or we have to know where it is and how to access it (written in a folder somewhere? On the Intranet? Or on a website? Which one?). Then the filing system must be functioning so that we can find it (the last person who used the folder with guidelines didn't put it back on the shelf, or the Internet is down, or I can't get access to a computer as they all being used, or there is no 3G in the hospital so my mobile phone won't work).

Once we have located the guideline, we need to understand it in the way the author intended and then we have to choose to follow it! The guideline may have required advance explanation and should be written clearly so that a new user can follow all the steps it involves. Examples of these rule-based processes might also include care pathways, care bundles, and checklists.

When drafting these it must be very clear which information is an action (and who will need to complete this, and is there a time frame for that action?), and which information is included just for educational purposes. The idea is for these structured written resources is to make it easy for people to do the right thing, not to frustrate them by being ambiguous, unclear, or bureaucratic. These tools should be clearly conceived and then tested with a pilot group for usability. The key question to ask is, does this decision-making tool actually help make the decision we need to make?

Once we have initiated our treatment, how should we document our actions? How will the next person who is reading the notes know whether the action has been completed? Does a tick mean 'I've started that process' or 'I've finished it'? It is, of course, not enough merely to send off a blood test; it is the interpretation of the results in the context of the patient and his or her condition that is key. Who will be responsible for that? How will that person know that it is for them to do this? How will that information be shared? Who might need to know? How will the next person on the next shift know who needs to know?

Clearly just having a guideline is not enough.

Let us move on to those cases where, for example, no matter how hard we try we cannot link things together to make a pattern that we recognize, or perhaps where we have exhausted our list of treatments but to no avail. We are now moving into the realms of creative decision making.

Creative decision making

In a non-acute setting we are more likely to be able to tap into creative solutions. It may be that we can use the principle that many heads are better than one. By calling a multidisciplinary meeting we will be able to bring in ideas from different perspectives. By convening a group of experts (e.g. a group of consultants, or a group of matrons, or a group of band 7s who all lead a team) they can share their combined experience (at a guess, on average 20 years of experience per person) to generate a new solution. Of course innovation must also happen safely (include lots of planning sessions, piloting, informed consent, peer review, product testing, etc.).

Any change always produces different responses in different people. There are early adopters who lap up anything new, a middle cohort who support a critical mass of opinion, and a few stragglers who prefer to leave things as they have always been. Some innovations that have happened within a theatre setting in my career jump to mind include laparoscopic cholecystectomy, the laryngeal mask, new anaesthetic machines and ventilators, total intravenous anaesthesia with propofol and remifentanil and enhanced recovery. In this list alone we have new techniques, new equipment, new drugs, and new ways of working, all of which began as one person's idea, which have been adopted and are now routine.

There are of course times when we are forced to be creative; for example, when a routine solution or piece of equipment fails in the middle of a procedure. What do we do when an emergency sneaks up in a routine setting?

As an overview of clinical decision making, I have constructed Figure 3.3 to allow us to visualize the complexity involved. Considering the complexity involved in decision making, it is not surprising that we make errors.

What style of decision making do you usually use? Are you aware of the pitfalls that you fall into? How will you identify your own hot spots and make them safer?

Routine becomes an emergency

We have talked about the challenges of 'transitioning' from a routine setting to one where an unexpected emergency has arisen. The first challenge—having been able to identify that the situation has changed—is to share this with the team ('This is now an emergency!') and to generate a shared situational assessment ('What do we think the problem is?').

Once we have identified the emergency we can use the same decision-making methods that we have already discussed: rule-based if an appropriate SOP (standard operating procedure) exists, recognition-primed if we need a speedy response and we have experience of the situation, option generation and creative if we have more time or because it is something completely new.

The tricky bit in this setting is where we admit to ourselves that things are not going as we had hoped or that we have missed something or the condition has deteriorated even though the patient was an inpatient and we have taken our eye off the ball. The part where most people seem to make poor decisions is our readiness to admit to ourselves that our mental model needs to change (see Figure 3.4).

Let us move to the final category of non-clinical decisions.

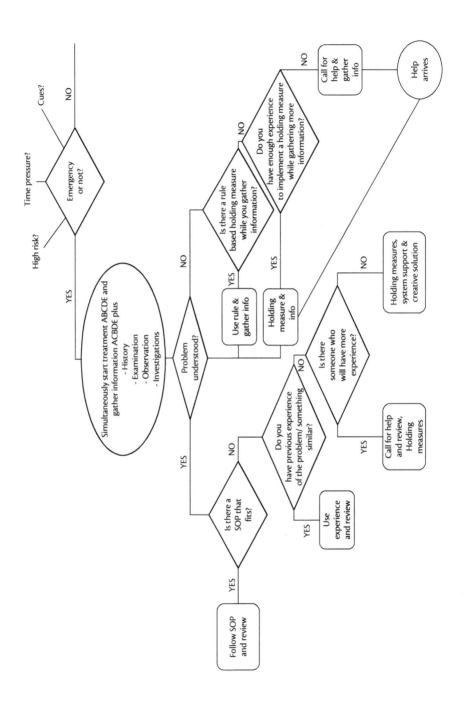

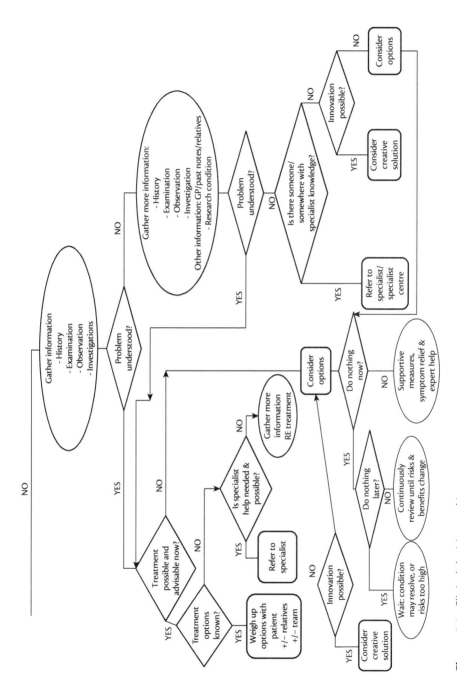

Figure 3.3 Clinical decision making.

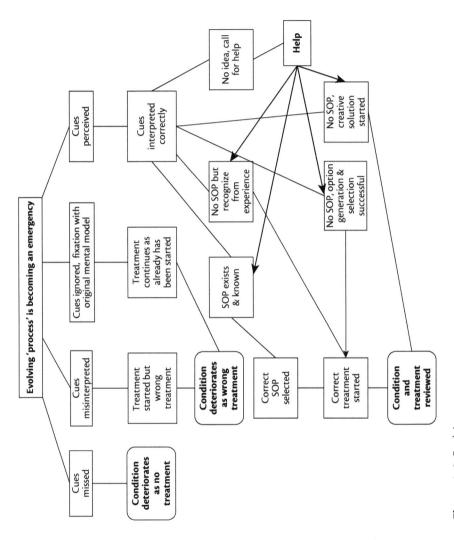

Figure 3.4 Evolving emergency.

Non-clinical decisions in a healthcare setting

If we start to explore the range of decisions that fall into this category we can start to get a feel for the enormous variety of decisions that we are grouping together under one heading. I am going to include all the decisions that are not directly about the care of one individual patient. Some of them certainly have clinical implications.

As I list some examples I want you to imagine which of the four decision-making categories might be most suitable for each (option generation, rule-based, recognition-primed, creative). I would also like you to consider *who* should be included in the group that is making the decision. Ask yourself: *how* they would be:

Dealing with an incident that might be a never event?

Deciding the outcome of a disciplinary hearing?

Planning how to spend next year's budget at an inter-departmental level?

Deciding how to manage the sickness rates on a particular ward?

Deciding which equipment to procure for a new surgical technique?

Deciding how to expand the catering service to increase its capacity?

Deciding who to appoint for a new role at interview?

Planning a five-year strategic plan?

Deciding how to cope with a complaint?

Deciding how to deal with a predicted overspend of £1 million by the end of the financial year?

Deciding what to do when the hospital is full and there is a queue of ambulances at the door of the emergency department?

Deciding what to do when there is a massive IT failure across the entire organization?

Deciding how to improve patient safety?

Planning how to improve networks between primary and secondary care?

Deciding what to do when asbestos is suddenly located within an area that was having building works?

Planning the contract cleaning services for the organization for the next year?

Dealing with your receptionist in a general practice after repeated complaints about her from patients?

Deciding how to hit targets (could be primary or secondary care)?

Planning educational initiatives for a particular staff group?

Deciding how to improve patient experience?

Deciding how to change the system for TTOs (drugs to take home, to take off) with pharmacy?

Planning a governance system?

Deciding how to expand a research department?

Planning how to increase the market share of what is being commissioned?

Running a monthly meeting?

The labour ward is full and they are phoning to see if they can 'go onto divert'. Will you?

The same principles apply. If there is an appropriate policy/guideline/SOP we should use that where appropriate. We will generally have more time than we think we have. It is the perceived risk and time pressure that will still influence how we make decisions. Those situations where we perceive the risk to be high we might be more likely to use a recognition-primed response and yet this may not be the best response. I ask you to remain aware in these settings of *how* you are making decisions (we are back to the concept of metacognition: thinking about how we think). I want you to remain aware of what is influencing your decision making and therefore how your decision making might be flawed.

There are whole books on strategic decision making so here I will simply give a few ideas to consider.

Six thinking hats

I want to introduce one of the classic concepts (although it still divides opinion): De Bono's six thinking hats.[9] This is a type of option-generation method to be used by a team. There are six differently coloured hats, representing six ways of thinking. Presented with any given problem, team members put on different hats to examine the problem from different perspectives and come up with a final solution.

This method takes some time to learn but it can generate a very thorough exploration of a possible solution.

The **white hat** represents logic, analysis, and data. This hat is about gathering information and facts. Do we have all the information we need? Do we have enough historical data to indicate trends? What other information might we need to know and how will we get it? This hat lets us remain objective and analytical.

The **red hat** represents emotions, gut instincts, and intuition. It allows us to consider the emotional responses both in the room and those that the decision might generate in others. It is much more about perceptions and subjectivity, and about trying to understand emotional responses in others.

The **black hat** represents the pessimistic approach. This is the time for the Mood Hoover! This calls for skepticism and cynicism; where will the plan fail? It is important to identify these problems now before you embark on the decision/plan so that you can strengthen the plan. It includes risk assessment and critical thinking. It is designed to identify any problems that the decision may cause.

The **yellow hat** represents a return to sunshine and optimism! It examines the best-case scenario and all of the benefits that would arise from the given decision or plan. It should also lift spirits, something that might be essential after the team has worn the black hat!

The **green hat** represents creativity and letting go. This is an opportunity to let the creative juices flow. It is time for ingenuity, innovation, brainstorming, for generating new ideas which can be expressed without fear of criticism.

The **blue hat** represents a more structured approach to thinking about the big picture. Here we start to consider the process as a whole and look at everything wearing the other hats has brought to bear on our current plan or decision. This is where we pull it all together. Have we covered it all?

You need a chair/coordinator to introduce each stage and clarify the sort of responses wearing each hat should encourage. They decide when enough ideas have been generated and then move the team on to wearing the next hat. At the end of the session you can be confident that the problem or the plan or the decision has been examined from every available perspective, all flaws considered, and all contingencies covered.

A variation on this theme is to consider the decision from the perspective of a different type of person, for example, a patient, a doctor, a nurse, etc.

Black swan

The black swan is not really a model; it is more a conceptual technique that we have already mentioned in the clinical setting. The black swan tells you to expect the unexpected and explore all the 'what ifs?' For example, when we have switched over to our new electronic patient record, *what if* the whole IT system failed?

SWOT

I am sure you have heard of SWOT analysis, looking at the strengths, weaknesses, opportunities, and threats of a given issue. This is often performed by dividing a sheet of flip chart paper into four sections (with or without sticky notes! And yes, I am poking fun at myself!) This analysis lets us explore how we can play to our strengths, to reinforce any areas where there might be weaknesses, where we can maximize our opportunities, and be aware of any problems that might derail what we are trying to achieve.

This technique has been around for a very long time. It can be used for both personal and team issues. I have seen half-hearted attempts at it that don't really achieve very much but I have also seen it used to great effect. It was originally introduced to help improve team understanding of their objectives. It is helpful to think about the questions you want to ask in advance.

Pugh matrix / grid analysis

This is also be known as multi-attribute utility theory, and can be quite useful if you need to weigh up a few options.[10]

Let us suppose there is a new role coming up in your department (the departmental lead, for example). You are interested in the role but it would mean changing other parts of what you do. There may also be changes in your hours and the days you have to work which might affect your home life. There should be more money in the new role but also more responsibility. There is a tricky colleague who may be particularly challenging to manage.

I have included a grid as Figure 3.5. Please look at this now. It is worth copying it onto a sheet of paper. This is much easier if you do it as I take you through it.

Across the top we write down the options that we want to weigh up (there can be more than two options). In this case the options might be column 2 (stay in current role) and column 3 (take on lead role). Down the left-hand side list all

	Weighting	Stay in current		Take the lead myself	
	1	2a	2b	3a	3b
Childcare change	x	0	0x	−1	−x
Tim the Tricky	y	0	0y	−1	−y
Money	z	0	0z	+2	+2z
Tim the Tricky gets the lead	a	−2	−2a	+2	+2a
......	......	......	......	......	......
......	......	......	......	......	......
Total	x + y + z + a......= 100		0 + 0 + 0 − 2a + ... =		−x − y + 2z + 2a +...... =

Figure 3.5 Our example mapped on to a Pugh matrix.[9]

the components that may change if we take the new role (for example, these could include give up clinic on Tuesday morning, change childcare arrangements, more money, more responsibility, dealing with Tim the Tricky, opens doors for future promotions, and so on). Feel free to add extras to this hypothetical example.

In columns 2a and 3a we are going to decide how much of each change would occur in the different settings. We assign it a numerical value. We assign 0 if that option wouldn't affect the component on the left. We give it +1 if it would make it better, and −1 if it would make it worse. (It is possible to also use +2 if it would be a lot better, and −2 if it would be a lot worse.)

We now need to decide how important each of these changes might be to us. We are going to give each activity a weighting and we are going to put the weighting in column 1. We are going to give each of these changes a number, to represent how important they are to you. There are different ways to score the weighting but I like to use 100 points as a total. These 100 points must be allocated between the rows so that you have used all of the 100 points but no more. This forces you to consider how bad it is to deal with Tim the Tricky versus changing childcare arrangements.

There is now a bit of maths. Apologies!

Multiply column 2a by column 1 and write the result in column 2b.

Multiply column 3a by column 1 and write the result in column 3b.

Now add up all the answers for column 2b to give a total at the bottom.

Add up all the answers for column 3b to give a total at the bottom.

Have a look at the scores. The one with the highest score is the winner. The interesting bit comes when you look at the result. How do you feel? Are you pleased or disappointed? Are you surprised? Would you like to change the result? Would that decision pass the champagne test (i.e. if you got the job, would you celebrate?)? The reaction can be equally important as the numerical value.

There are many other tools available that can be helpful, and I have simply covered a few of the common ones. Now I want to consider the final part of decision making, the part that involves the entire team.

Team or joint decision making

It can be hard enough to gather the correct information in the time allowed, having weighed up the risk and employed the correct decision-making method to help us to find the optimum solution when we are working on our own. But what happens when we have a team all perceiving different information at different rates with different perspectives and values and past experiences, all assessing risk differently against different benchmarks—how are we going to unite them in the decision-making process?

It is because we work with large numbers of people and must move information between them, process that information and decide what to do about it, that I want to spend a bit of time concentrating on the 'team' aspect of decision making. I am not talking about a stable team in the traditional sense, hence the term 'joint decision making' rather than 'team decision making' may be more accurate.

It may be a joint decision made by a patient and a clinician. The joint decision may involve a group of people in an emergency setting around a bedside. The joint decision may be made by a group of one type of professionals in a meeting (e.g. nursing handover, consultant meeting). A mixture of professionals could make the joint decision (e.g. an oncology MDT). Clinicians and managers may make the joint decision. Primary and secondary care may make joint decisions. Healthcare and social care may make joint decisions. We hope that our patient and their relatives will feel that they are included in a joint decision-making process.

We talked in Chapter 2 about creating a shared mental model and in this chapter about how this needs to build towards a shared situational assessment. We need to agree on the problem definition.

The first key step is accurately gathering and sharing the information (see Box 3.1). The way this information needs to be shared depends on which of the four settings we are in (emergency/routine/unexpected/non-clinical). In an

> ## Box 3.1 A recap
>
> *Remember some of the simple techniques to underpin information sharing*
>
> ◆ *Read back—when we ask someone to repeat something back to us to confirm the information transfer has taken place.*
>
> ◆ *Avoid of pronouns.*
>
> ◆ *Cross check—when we ask someone to check something with us, we ask, 'what is this?' to avoid confirmation bias.*
>
> ◆ *Active identification.*
>
> ◆ *Beware of assumptions—check that you and the team have the same understanding of the language you are using.*

emergency setting it may be that the information is fed to the leader who may ultimately make the decisions but with team input when time allows or at key stages throughout the process.

When more time is available, it is possible to use a much more collaborative approach. We can take time to elicit everyone's thoughts and to listen to them. It may be that a more junior member of the team (depending on the perceived hierarchy gradient), or a more introverted team member with a reflective learning style, may need longer to prepare before they feel able to contribute their idea. This is worth waiting for as it might well be that this person then delivers a real gem of an idea or offers a brand new perspective that has not yet been considered. It is important to value everyone's input and not to let 'status' or position in a hierarchy inhibit anyone contributing.

How are you going to make sure that you give everyone in your team a voice? Who will find it most difficult to speak up?

First, I want to make a couple of suggestions of things to avoid. I tend to avoid what is sometimes called 'death by circle'. Taking it in turn to speak simply by going around the room will not give room for the differences in personalities and thinking styles to arise. Some people become more worried about their turn approaching than they are about the problem they are trying to solve. I also tend to avoid naming people and putting them on the spot. If they are of a more reflective persuasion, this may induce a 'bunny in the headlights' moment.

Instead, I would open the discussion up and wait for people to speak when they are ready. If you know the group, perhaps try to catch the eye of someone you know to be more extrovert or more confident on the topic and try to encourage him or her to speak first to start the ball rolling.

If there is a history of conflict in the group or a steep hierarchy gradient, consider collecting ideas on sticky notes and put them up randomly and anonymously on a flipchart. Be encouraging and use your enthusiasm to lift the energy in the room.

(For those of you who are by now squirming, I realize that not everyone can run a successful option-generation session. When we discuss team working in more detail, it may be that you will recognize those in your group who may be comfortable in these kinds of session. I promise that if you identify these people and encourage them to talk (and to take turns listening) you will get better results than using the 'death by circle' method. It is best to have a mixture of introverts and extroverts, but we need to make sure that one or two individuals don't dominate the group. If you have a room full of people who all like 'death by circle' what might the dangers of that be?)

In a positive decision-making episode we need people to feel able to put forward opposing viewpoints. If people disagree in this setting it improves the breadth of option generation and makes for more creative/innovative ideas. (We don't want to get stuck in 'group think' or in hero-worshipping mode.) However, once different ideas are produced we either have to try them all or select which one we going to opt for and try to take the team with us on that decision!

The next question is: how is the group going to decide to make the decision?

Will the leader make the decision, or the team, or both? Will everyone have to agree (consensus)? Or will a majority opinion be good enough? If accepting a majority opinion how will you know you have a majority and how big a majority does it have to be? Would it involve a vote or some other method? And if a voting method were to be used would it be open and visible or anonymous? Would the process have to happen anyway, even if the group doesn't want it? If this group proposes an idea, can it go forward or does it have to be approved by someone else? Are there sufficient funds to support all of the options?

When you work in a group making a decision, do you ever spend a few minutes considering how you worked together that day? Do you think 'how well did we do that? What can we learn from it?' If I ask this question, the replies have ranged from, 'no, I never even thought about it', to a more defensive 'we don't have time', sometimes accompanied by an unspoken 'don't you know how busy we are!' (see Box 3.2).

Box 3.2 Soap-box moment

Yes, we are incredibly pressed for time and resource poor. I am fully aware that our bed occupancy in some organizations is currently at 110 per cent, meaning we are having to turn things around so that we have more than one patient in a bed on a single day. (The ideal is about 85 per cent, so no wonder we are making errors when under this sort of pressure.)

The very reason that we are under this pressure is why it is even more important that we use our time and resources and make decisions wisely. You wouldn't dream of letting a surgeon loose with a scalpel without first training her to use it. Why should we assume that we are naturally skilled at making decisions, especially when we will be under some kind of pressure? If we acknowledge that we will not all be instantly gifted at this then surely we should be training people how to do it well, and trying to improve our own capabilities. If we know that our decisions affect the treatments of our patients and some of our decisions are lifesaving and life changing, why are we not paying more attention to these skills? Why are we not teaching all our medical students, nursing students, AHP students across the organization to our GPs, consultants, consultant nurses, matrons, executive members, boards, and clinical commissioning groups how to work together to make good decisions?

The next time you are coming towards the end of an MDT or any sort of meeting (and don't get me started on how many meetings are actually useful in the NHS), perhaps you could spend a couple of minutes looking at how it ran. I want to share with you the advanced team decision model (ATDM) that was developed by Zsambok.[1,11] This model contains ten key behaviours that they found are possessed by high-performing teams (see Figure 3.6). These ten behaviours can be categorized into three groups under the broad headings of strong team identity, team thinking, and team self-monitoring. It is worth emphasizing that this model is used for those who are planning rather than in the middle of actually doing (i.e. strategic rather than operational). It is suitable for any sort of meeting or an MDT but would not be suitable for a team in the middle of managing a cardiac arrest.

Imagine a meeting that you either chair or that you attend as we consider this in more detail.

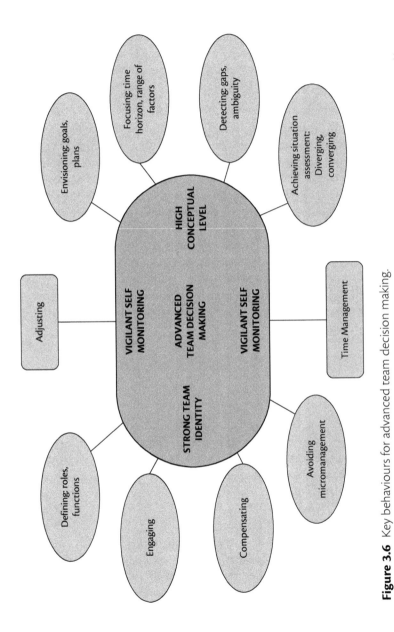

Figure 3.6 Key behaviours for advanced team decision making.

Reproduced with permission from Zsambok, CE, Klein, G, Kyne, MM, and Klinger, DW (1992). *Advanced team decision making: A developmental model.* (Prepared under Contract MDA903-90-C-0117 for U.S. Army Research Institute for the Behavioral and Social Sciences) Fairborn, OH: Klein Associates Inc. Copyright © 2015 Applied Research Associates, Inc.

Strong team identity

Within the team, people need to understand who is doing what and how that serves a function within the whole. (Can each of your team answer the following questions: why am I here? What is my role? What am I expected to contribute? How does that fit into the big picture?) They also need to want to be there and want to contribute. (How are you going to engage the less willing members and how are you going to motivate them?) They need to be able to cover for each other's weaknesses or absence. (How will you know where the weaknesses are?) The team should not be stifled by micro-management but instead given the freedom to flourish. (How will you balance nudging the process in the right direction and gently steering whilst encouraging new ideas?)

Team thinking

The team needs to have a shared understanding of why they are there. (Have you ever been to a meeting and wondered 'what are we trying to do here?') The team needs to develop shared goals and a shared direction of travel. (How will you know whether everyone has the same idea of where you are aiming?) There needs to be a shared understanding of both focus and the scope of the contributory factors that are to be considered. (How will the focus and the boundaries be defined?) The team needs to be able to identify gaps. (What are we missing here?) The team needs to reduce duplication and clarify any ambiguity. (Which bits might be clear to us, but not to all of our patients/staff? What assumptions have we made?) They need to have a shared situational awareness (consider using SHEEP as a framework to have the conversation for situational awareness—what is the problem? So what? Which systems/guidelines/SOPs/information do we need? Who do we need? Who will do what? Where do we need to do it? What equipment do we need? Will I have the right expertise for this? How full is my bucket? What next?).

Self-monitoring

I tend to rant when I come to this last category. This is the part where we actually monitor how well we are doing something as well as actually doing it. It is the admission that simply doing it is not enough; we really care how well we are doing it. We need to learn to adjust, continuously making little tweaks and improvements, as an integral part of the process itself. It is self-monitoring that enables continuous improvement.

We are also aware of the timing of the task and the length of time in which we have to perform it. Someone will need to keep time for the planning and to keep track of the time once the process becomes operational.

Here is a list of examples that you can work through to identify the decision-making methods that might be most appropriate for some sample situations. A range of examples can be found below (see Example 3.5) and the answers that I thought were most appropriate are offered (see Example 3.6) with a discussion so that you can compare your thinking to mine. (It doesn't mean I'm right!) If you get stuck, try using Figure 3.2 to follow the possible pathways.

Example 3.5 Scenarios for practising decision making

1. Orthopaedic: a patient with a high body-mass index and multiple morbidities who would benefit from a knee replacement. Do they need to lose weight first? Do they need to be optimized first? Should we operate soon or later?

2. Anaesthetic: a patient who needs an anaesthetic. Will it be spinal/regional/GA? Which analgesics? Which anti-emetics?

3. Pre-operative antibiotics: which one for this procedure? And when should it be given?

4. Obstetric/midwifery: interpretation of a foetal trace.

5. Critical care: interpretation of an ECG waveform or $EtCO_2$ waveform (for non-clinical readers, this is the level of carbon dioxide released at the end of an exhalation).

6. Cardiac arrest: first diagnosing cardiac arrest, then starting treatment, and then the 4Hs and 4Ts.

7. GP: taking a telephone history and deciding whether the patient should be seen or stay at home or simply be treated without being seen.

8. Emergency general surgery: bleeding laparotomy, do we pack it and wait?

9. Renal: starting CAPD (continuous ambulatory peritoneal dialysis) or dialysis, and when?

10. MDT: a patient has a diagnosis of cancer. They need surgery, chemotherapy, and radiotherapy, but in which order?

11. Using a care bundle.

12. Dealing with a failing trainee.

13. A patient with chest pain.

14. Anaesthesia/PITU: the induction of a seriously unwell, emergency paediatric patient in a DGH.

15. Anaesthesia: inventing TIVA or the laryngeal mask airway?

16. Whether to start using a new innovation.

17. How to deal with staff sickness.

18. Intensive care: can we just start organ support or do we need the diagnosis so that we can start the correct treatment?

19. Intensive care: the first person to use remifentanil for sedation.

20. A patient with a stroke.

21. Theatre: how to perform a WHO checklist? Do we just go through the motions, or are we creative and tailor it to our specific situation and use it as part of briefing process that we really own, and identify our hot spots, and highlight our team working?

22. Theatre teams: stable versus rotating.

23. Discontinuing CPR.

Example 3.6 Scenarios for practising decision making: Discussion

1. Orthopaedic: a patient with a high body-mass index and multiple morbidities who would benefit from a knee replacement. Do they need to lose weight first? Do they need to be optimized first? Should we operate sooner or later?

   My thoughts are that this is a case of option generation and choice. It may be that there will be an element of rule-based decision making in some organizations where guidelines may be in place.

2. Anaesthetic: a patient who needs an anaesthetic. Will it be spinal/regional/GA? Which analgesics? Which anti-emetics?

   Option generation and choice.

3. Pre-operative antibiotics: which one for this procedure? And when should it be given?

   Rule-based. There should be evidence-based information that is encompassed into a guideline that has been agreed by (and kept up to date with) microbiologists and theatre staff. The rules need to be known and, I would suggest, easily accessible, or even better, clearly displayed as an up-to-date resource.

4. Obstetric/midwifery: interpretation of a foetal trace.

   I think this is a tricky one. Of course, there are rules that people are taught about interpreting traces but there is also a large amount of experience required. I have witnessed several senior clinicians in heated debate about the interpretation of a CTG (cardiotocograph). It is something that is signed regularly throughout a patient's labour. It has medico-legal implications. Whilst we might like to think of it as rule based, I think it has a large degree of recognition-primed. (I'd be happy to debate that with you if we were able to talk to each other!)

5. Critical care: interpretation of an ECG waveform or $EtCO_2$ waveform.

   As above, we are trained on courses or from textbooks and other sources about how to interpret these waveforms. We like to think that our interpretation would be standardized and this would all be rule-based decision making but again, I think there is a large degree of recognition-primed interpretation.

6. Cardiac arrest: first diagnosing cardiac arrest, then starting treatment, and then the 4Hs and 4Ts.

I have thought about this one for a long time. Assuming we are the first responder, initially we l have to recognize that the patient might have arrested (recognition-primed). Next we have to confirm our suspicions (rule-based— ABC—open airway, confirm no breaths, and no pulse for 10 seconds (except in hypothermia)). Start treatment (rule-based as per ALS guidelines) and within that rule-based option generation (4Hs and 4Ts).

7. GP: taking a telephone history and deciding whether the patient should be seen or stay at home or simply be treated without being seen.

This seems to be happening increasingly as primary care faces more challenges. It is a lot of responsibility to triage by phone. We have discussed how much information is picked up non-verbally and we are now expecting our doctors to diagnose without being able to communicate non-verbally and without any physical signs or cues. You can tell a lot about how unwell someone is by looking at them. You can't see them on the phone. We are expecting our GPs to generate options and make choices under challenging conditions.

8. Emergency general surgery: bleeding laparotomy: do we pack it and wait?

Weighing up risks and benefits: option generation and choice. Realizing that you should be considering those options and taking time out: you could argue that this comes down to experience and gut instinct (recognition-primed) or that it is rule-based ('first, do no harm').

9. Renal: starting CAPD or dialysis, and when?

Option generation and choice.

10. MDT: a patient has a diagnosis of cancer. They need surgery, chemotherapy, and radiotherapy, but in which order?

I have heard that this debate is sometimes full of differing opinions but I hope that this generates great option generation and choice.

11. Using a care bundle.

I suspect this is another one that could cause much discussion. Care bundles are devised to be rule based. They are supposed to be evidenced based. They are supposed to be time saving and have a built-in safety net that helps to act as an aide memoire so we don't forget key steps in a process.

*However, the quality of the care bundles I have experienced is very variable. A care bundle needs to be well publicized so that people know when to use it. It needs to be accessible so that with almost no effort it can be found. (**We need to make it easy for people to do the right thing**.) It needs to be simple to understand without any prior training: we have very high staff turnover (e.g. trainees rotating every 3–6 months). It must be clear which parts are for information only and which parts are actions that must be completed.*

*One of the decisions here is the decision whether or not to use the care bundle. If it is felt to be out of date, difficult to use, reliant on a poor evidence base, poorly written, ambiguous, or too long, then the decision may be to **not** use the guideline or care bundle. This is a complex decision of whether or not to use a work-around. It is partly cultural, influenced by time constraints (and whether it was quick to use last time!), and heavily influenced by the perceived usefulness of the tool. There are also influences such as lack of expert buy-in and engagement, change management, and the ownership of the process.*

My personal thoughts are that this takes us back to using the fast system 1, and making an overall gut decision about whether we think the care bundle will be useful for us/our patient. So whilst we should be following a rule-based decision, we are actually using recognition-primed decision making, although we might justify in the cold light of day using system 2 and logical option generation and choice.

Again, I'm happy to be challenged on that one!

12. **Dealing with a failing trainee.**

This situation is also incredibly complex. Of course, we would like to think that we have rules in place that mean we should easily identify someone who is falling below standard. However, my experience is that the situation is rather more complicated. There may well be a list of competencies that are not being achieved, making it easy to reach a conclusion based on rules, but what if it is just a feeling that something isn't quite right? The majority of failing trainees do not have a problem with their knowledge or their skills but instead with their non-technical skills. It is harder to recognize these deficiencies in the first place as they are often not assessed, and then hard to analyse exactly what the problem is.

Is it a lack of ability to prioritize and filter? Is it a time-management issue? Is it an organizational issue? Is it rooted in team working or sharing information? Does the problem lie in the ability to generate a shared mental model and team decision making? Is it a lack of assertiveness or the desire to run a very steep hierarchy? Is it an inability to cope with more than one set of data at a time? Is the individual not suited to cope with the stress or the time pressure or workload that is required of them in a particular specialty? Is it how he or she interacts with other staff or with patients? What if the individual is not aware of his or her own shortcomings?

These issues are very difficult to analyse. I have yet to see a rulebook that covers for all of these eventualities. I would say that some decisions in these settings are recognition primed but with enough experience and hard work there can be option generation and choice. This problem may also need creative solutions if there is something new discovered, but by the time this stage is reached, expertise should have been sought.

All this means I have hedged my bets and opted for all four types of decision making in this setting!

13. A patient with chest pain.

    Rule-based with targets for door to needle time.

14. Anaesthesia/PITU: the induction of a seriously unwell, emergency paediatric patient in a DGH without its own PITU.

    This requires joint decision making between the two centres. Ideally ahead of time there will have been education and decisions made between the experts at both centres. In an ideal world, there will be a protocol agreed which all of the consultants have been involved in and have agreed to (this will involve option generation, choice, and shared decision making).

    The generation of this SOP (standard operating procedure/guideline/protocol) is designed to relieve the pressure in the heat of the emergency. It allows for the use of rule-based decision making in the stressful situation of a paediatric emergency. The stress levels are driven by potential lack of familiarity or feeling at the edge of someone's comfort zone. It may be 'luck' that the person in the DGH who is working that day has specialist paediatric expertise, or it may be 'unlucky' that they are one of the less-confident members of the department. We have to make allowances if it is the latter. Of course, in our perfect world everyone would be confident and competent at everything. In reality, the truth is that we all have our strengths and preferences and ideally we can play to those. But at times we will have to cover things that push us to our limits, and occasionally beyond.

15. Anaesthesia: inventing TIVA or the laryngeal mask airway.

    Without innovation, how do we move forward? But how do we know change brings with it improvement?

    I have chosen the use of TIVA and the LMA as these are two landmark innovations that have completely changed anaesthetic practice within my career.

My thoughts lie firstly with the inventors. What sort of decision was it when they decided to try a new technique or tried a new way of doing something? I am making an assumption here but I think there is a combination of creative decisions mixed with option generation for all of the possibilities that are tried.

16. Whether to start using a new innovation.

*If we then consider the next steps, how do others adopt a brand new idea? How do they decide it is a **good** idea? When do they decide it is OK, and how to they make that decision?*

There are different phases of change. There is usually a group of early adopters who begin using a new technique or device soon after it is released.

As the innovation is publicized via journals, conferences, and by word of mouth, its use gathers momentum. The decisions here I think are largely option generation and choice; weighing up the evidence for the new technique but considering how to adapt it to one's own practice probably involves some creative decision-making too.

17. How to deal with staff sickness.

I have seen a wide range of approaches to this in my time in the NHS. There is the entirely rule-based approach: what does the policy say? We will follow that to the letter.

I have also seen what people describe as a 'common-sense' approach. I know which of my staff are reliable and which of them are 'swinging the lead'.

Where does common sense fit in with decision making? Is it a logical weighing-up of different options, or is it intuitive and a sense of 'you just know what to do' (recognition-primed)?

18. Intensive care: can we just start organ support, or do we need the diagnosis so that we can start the correct treatment?

I chose this dilemma as it was something that a very eminent consultant put to me when I was training. I had admitted a patient and had provided three organ support (ventilation, cardiovascular, and renal), but I didn't really have a clear diagnosis. I had in fact made decisions that were within my experience. I could decide to start each of those supportive measures and I knew how to carry them out, but during that time I had not spent the addition brain power on what was actually the underlying condition. I had despatched investigations to try to gather more information to help me understand what this condition might be, but I could not use my pattern recognition to piece it together.

The consultant asked me 'how can you treat someone if you don't know what you are treating?' I was simply putting in a holding measure (three organ support).

I was reminded of a trip I made to the vet (about 20 years ago so I'm sure it won't hold true now!). My cat had developed a sort of skin condition. The vet couldn't decide between two diagnostic options and so suggested an injection of antibiotics and an injection of steroids, saying that one of those should work!

Returning to my ITU consultant, I felt that he was correct but I found myself wondering. How could I decide on a diagnosis? I didn't have enough knowledge or experience yet on which to draw. I was comforted when it actually took a meeting of several consultants and a lively debate to make the decision on what to do.

19. Intensive care: the first person to use remifentanil for sedation.

    This involved taking a drug infusion that was gaining popularity in a theatre setting and making a creative decision to see if it would work in another setting, but I'm sure the options and risks were carefully considered too and that there was also an element of choice within the decision.

20. A patient with a stroke.

    Rule-based.

21. Theatre: how to perform a WHO checklist? Do we just go through the motions or are we creative and tailor it to our specific situation, and use it as part of briefing process that we really own. Do we use it to identify our hot spots and highlight our team working?

    I have the utmost respect for Atul Gawande's[12–14] work that has led to the implementation of the WHO checklist in theatre across the UK and in many places worldwide. I do not have the same degree of respect for those people who are either casual and sloppy with their checklist, or completely maverick and think they are too good for it. And yes, both attitudes were initially common. I think over time there has been a gradual culture change.

    The effectiveness of the checklist depends on its weakest link—and that is the person using it.

    So what type of decision is it when you decide whether or not you are going to follow the rules?

    One of the trendy rebuttals for change currently is 'where's the evidence?' People mutter this as almost as a reflex; I suspect it is a fast system 1 response.

However, this could not be used with Gawande's work because the pilot across three very different hospitals showed clear evidence of positive change.

The next excuse can sometimes involve something about impinging on someone's 'professionalism' or 'autonomy'. How professional is it to bypass a WHO guideline?

We all have a different approach to change. Is it that this change somehow threatens something and if so, what? If I was playing devil's advocate I might suggest that there is a power play involved. Perhaps someone who considers him or herself to be at the top of the food chain is now having to conform and do as he or she is asked? Surely that can't be it!

There must be a logical system 2 response with option generation and choice as to why someone would ignore a mandate? So what might be the underlying reason for a work around being used in place of an entirely sensible practice?

Another rebuttal is that the checklist stops people thinking. For me, this is the crux regarding how we use the checklist. It comes back to not the checklist itself but to how we interact with it. If it becomes a brainless box-ticking exercise then it loses its power.

We need to engage our grey cells when we go through the checklist procedure. I know there are some things that have infuriated people and have hence damaged the embedding process. For example, if you have an eye list, I believe is physically impossible to lose over 500 mls of blood. So asking this question about every eye patient is illogical and unhelpful. There are other lists where blood loss is incredibly rare, so remove that question from the list. If people believe you are wasting their time, particularly as most theatres are time poor and under high workload pressures, it will trigger frustration. This may, in turn, make committing an error more likely!

In some theatres there may need to be additions to the list; for example, a paediatrician might not be needed for every list but they would be an important consideration for an emergency caesarean section!

I know that this common-sense approach is gaining momentum.

22. Theatre teams: stable versus rotating.

Continuing with the theatre theme, I want to consider how an organization decides whether to have static theatre scrub teams or ones that rotate.

If Michael West[15] were here, he would tell you that the argument is very strongly in favour of stable teams.

It is easier to work with someone that you know. You understand each other more easily and should be able to communicate better. You will have developed *your roles and have better role clarity. You will be familiar with how each other like to work (**H**).*

*You will know how you like your **E**nvironment laid out (which side someone likes to operate, where she wants the scrub side to set up, where he wants the stacking system, and so on).*

*You will know which kit is preferred (**E**quipment).*

*You will learn one another's strengths and capabilities. You might know if someone has something stressful going on at home which is filling his or her bucket. You might pick up on cues more quickly if someone is struggling or out of his or her depth (**P**).*

So the issue of whether to run a stable team to me is fairly easy to answer. It is a question of weighing up the options and making a choice.

I can understand that if you will have to cover the emergency theatre as part of your role that then you should spend time in different theatres to maintain a broad skill base, but surely you can rotate just one of the team at a time, leaving it relatively intact?

When I am told 'it just isn't possible, I am a glass full to overflowing', I am sure that in fact it is possible but we need to think harder to generate new solutions. Perhaps these would be creative decisions?

23. Discontinuing CPR.

It is a challenging time when a team has worked hard to try to resuscitate someone and there has been no progress. I wonder what factors might make you think, just a bit longer?

What if the patient is younger than you or is a child? What if he or she was fit and healthy previously with no pre-existing morbidities? What if a relative is watching you? What if a whole ward of people is watching you? What if something occurred to you that had not yet been tried?

Let's assume that we have tried everything. We have exhausted all the options from the ALS guidelines. It now seems hopeless, so what should we do?

This should be an example of shared decision making. The main options are whether to carry on or to stop, and this is a choice decision. But how are you going to make that choice? Are you going to wait for consensus (everyone has to agree), or go with majority votes, or can the team leader make that final decision, or does it default to someone who isn't even present (perhaps the consultant who is at home but it is 'their' patient)?

Key points (up to and including Chapter 3)

- Situational awareness can be separated into three components: perception, comprehension, and predicting a future state. (What? So what? What next?)

- We make sense of what we have perceived and turn it into a mental model.

- When working in a team it is important that the mental model is shared with and shared by the team members. (Remember commentating.)

- This shared mental model builds towards a team situational assessment or problem definition.

- Barriers to perception and comprehension include:

  - high workload,

  - time pressure,

  - perceived high risk,

  - stress,

  - fatigue,

  - biases (including expectation, confirmation, and environmental), and

  - task fixation.

- When building our mental model problems can arise due to:

  - missed cues,

  - misinterpreting cues, or

  - choosing to ignore cues,

  - incorrect risk assessment,

  - poor time judgement, or

  - a failure to update our mental model either when new information becomes available or when conditions change.

- It can be useful to do a quick run through SHEEP to help with situational awareness:

  - S—Which guideline/SOP are we using? Do we have all of the information we need?

- ♦ H—Who is doing what? How is that working? Is someone time keeping?

- ♦ E—Are we in the best place for what we are dealing with?

- ♦ E—Do we have all the kit that we need?

- ♦ P—How full is my bucket? Where is my focus?

♦ Once we have completed our situational assessment or problem definition we move on to ask 'what are we going to do about it?'

♦ There are four main types of decision-making process:[1,2]

- ♦ recognition-primed or intuitive,

- ♦ rule-based,

- ♦ option generation, and

- ♦ creative.

♦ How we decide which method suits the situation depends on time pressure, risk, and the novelty of the situation.

♦ The rule-based approach for emergencies exists to make life easier for healthcare staff. The resuscitation guidelines give us a shared experience and training of how to work as a team in these stressful settings. Once we have diagnosed a cardiac arrest we share that information with those around us, call for help to activate a larger team if required, and commence treatment as per the protocol.

♦ There is a stage of pattern recognition required in order to select a guideline or protocol. We can fail to identify the cues and triggers and hence fail to initiate the rule-based decisions.

♦ In a setting where there is a high level of risk and pattern recognition is possible, but in the absence of a rule-based solution, an experienced practitioner may opt for a recognition-primed response. This may require past experience, knowledge recall, and an almost automatic response to a situation. We need to be cautious in this setting with regards fixation error. Be aware of where your attention is directed and ask others for input when you have time. Ask yourself, 'what am I missing here and what else could this be?'

♦ When we have more time we can use an option-generation model such as DECIDE.

◆ When we face a novel problem, then the solution will potentially have to be creative. However, it may be that the problem is not novel to others so it is worth considering gathering more information, using cognitive aids, and pulling in other expertise.

◆ Making a decision is only the first step in a cycle. We should then continuously monitor that treatment or plan and review it. This is especially true in the light of new information.

◆ It is vital to update our mental model with new information.

◆ Please guard against the *assumption* that the diagnosis is definitely correct.

◆ We need to spend more time reviewing how we are making our decisions so that we can improve this skill.

References

1. Flin R, Crichton M. *Safety at the Sharp End; A Guide to Non-technical Skills*: Farnham: Ashgate, 2008.
2. Society Human Factors and Ergonomics. Training for Aviation Decision Making: The Naturalistic Decision Making Perspective. 39th Annual Meeting 1995; San Diego, Santa Monica, CA. The Human Factors and Erognomics Society.
3. Orasanu J. Crew Collaboration in Space: A Naturalistic Decision-Making Perspective. *Aviation, Space, and Environmental Medicine* 2005; 76(6 Suppl): B154–63.
4. Walters A. *Crew Resource Management is no Accident.* Wallingford: Aries, 2002.
5. Endsley M. Toward a Theory of Situation Awareness in Dynamic Systems. *Human Factors* 1995; 37: 32–64.
6. Klein G. Naturalistic Decision Making. *Human Factors* 2008; 50(3): 456–60.
7. Taleb NN. *The Black Swan: The Impact of the Highly Improbable*. London: Randon House, 2007.
8. Kahneman D. *Thinking Fast and Slow*. London: Allen Lane, 2011.
9. De Bono E. *Six Thinking Hats*. London: Penguin, 1985.
10. Pugh S. *Total Design: Integrated Methods for Successful Product Engineering*. Wokingham: Addison-Wesley, 1990.
11. Zsambok CE, Klein GA. *Naturalistic Decision Making*. Mahwah, NJ: Lawrence Erlbaum Associates, 1997.
12. Gawande A. The Checklist: If Something so Simple can Transform Intensive Care, What Else Can it Do? *New Yorker* 10 December 2007: 86–101.
13. Gawande A. Checklists for Success Inside the OR and Beyond: An Interview with Atul Gawanda, MD, FACS. Interview by Tony Peregrin. *Bulletin of the American College of Surgeons* 2010;95(5): 24–7.
14. Gawande A. *The Checklist Manifesto*. London: Picador, 2011.
15. Buttigieg SC, West MA, Dawson JF. Well-structured Teams and the Buffering of Hospital Employees from Stress. *Health Services Management Research* 2011;24(4): 203–12.

4

Conflict resolution and team development

Fear not those who argue but those who dodge.
Marie von Ebner-Eschenbach, 1830–1916

Conflict resolution

We spent the last chapter covering decision making and how we need to agree upon a shared mental model, but what happens when we don't agree?

The term *conflict* probably conjures up different images in different people. Take a moment to consider what comes to your mind. For some, it may bring up images of a generic war, or perhaps a more specific and current conflict. For others, something at work might spring to mind, and for others something at home. Conflict can be experienced in a range of ways from physical violence or shouting at one end of a spectrum, to silence, withdrawal, or avoidance. It is sometimes referred to as a process of 'naming, blaming, and shaming/claiming'.

Conflict can be defined as an 'unmet need'.

It can be considered under two headings: personal and substantive.

◆ Substantive conflict arises concerning processes, decisions, plans, actions, or ideas.

◆ Personal conflict, as the name implies, concerns individuals. It sometimes manifests itself as what is colloquially referred to as a personality clash. This emotionally charged interpersonal conflict is rarely helpful, nor is it a catalyst for change. It is something that requires resolving.

Interestingly, conflict is often viewed as a negative interaction. Substantive conflict does, however, have a place in moving things forward, promoting change and new ideas, and in option generation. It is acceptable to disagree with one another, but this ought to be done respectfully. We can take these differing views people hold and explore them to good effect. We can use these differences as a catalyst either

111

to understand a given situation more thoroughly or to understand each other better. This positive outcome does, of course, require some effort on both sides and some knowledge about how to try to reach the middle ground of consensus.

We know that unresolved conflict has a negative effect on the working environment and on the staff involved. We can end up stuck in something referred to as a conflict cycle where a previously unresolved conflict resurfaces at a subsequent interaction. When personal conflict arises it usually stems from one of both parties feeling that its needs are not being met. There is usually a perception that the other party has a difficult personality or is a tricky character or has an ulterior motive than the one he or she is claiming. The exchanges can potentially be emotionally charged and unresolved hostility can have a negative effect not only for the individuals directly involved but also for the team or department in which they work.

I am going to focus on resolving conflict in a work setting but some of what we cover will be along similar principles for conflict resolution in other settings.

Remember that if you are experiencing conflict at home, this will affect the 'work you'. Your bucket will already be fairly full before you come to work. Your stress levels will be high and you will be more likely to make a mistake at work, and making a mistake may be sufficient to make your bucket overflow.

A few examples of conflict at home

Perhaps you are facing a challenge with your partner. Divorce is incredibly common these days (one in three marriages ends in divorce in the general population, and in sections of healthcare, this rises to one in two). It may be that your conflict arises as your parents are now of an age that independent living for them is becoming a challenge. Perhaps you have teenage children: four of our children are teenagers and so I know how stressful living with teens can be. Perhaps you have problems juggling childcare with work, or your finances are stretched, or you have a sick relative, or a noisy neighbour, or you have been working long hours, or you are spending all your time studying for an exam and your 'significant other' feels rejected.

I urge you to think about resolving the conflict.

Work-based conflict

We have already explained that this may arise from either a personal or a substantive origin. Substantive conflict may be more easily managed. One of the ways to move personal conflict towards resolution can be to look for the substantive elements within the conflict. Personalized conflict may well have begun when previous substantive conflict was left unresolved.

We can consider conflict as having two contributory aspects: strength of feeling and willingness to cooperate. We may well have developed a preferred mode of dealing with conflict. I want you to consider how you usually behave in a conflict setting. Do you tend to hit it head on? Do you avoid it like the plague? Does it depend on whom it is with—'I'm scared of X, but I would handle it, if it was with someone more junior than me'? Or perhaps it depends on what it is about? Have a look at Figure 4.1.

We are back to something that we covered in Level One (pp. 72–82) but we are going to cover it in more depth here. Think about how each animal in the figure usually behaves.

I have chosen a bull to represent the metaphorical 'bull in a china shop'. This can also be referred to as the 'tank' or the aggressive approach to conflict. The strong sense of personal investment or pride and a lack of willingness to cooperate results in a victory for the bull and a loss for whoever the bull is up against— no other animal is thus represented here; the bull wins and that's that. This approach may occasionally be appropriate in an emergency or crisis situation where there is insufficient time for indecision or negotiation.

If we consider the box diagonally opposite the bull, the puppy wants to please people. This box represents a style of accommodation, or sometimes thought of as a person being something of a doormat. Whilst you might not fancy being a doormat, you might find it easier to think of yourself as a puppy. There can be a time to choose your battles. If you let the other party win on a topic that is not something you feel strongly about, you can effectively 'bank' a favour. (Beware, however, that karma is not a given!) Again I chose only one animal because once again, only one person can win in an interaction with a puppy, and it isn't the puppy! What is being represented here is 'I lose, you win'.

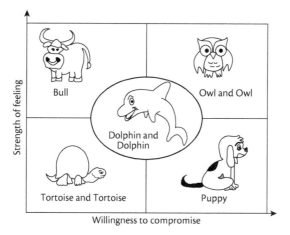

Figure 4.1 Conflict management styles.

If both parties would like to ignore or avoid the conflict I have chosen the obvious analogy of two tortoises but I could equally have chosen two ostriches. The problem with ignoring conflict is that the problems do not go away. An ongoing conflict cycle can ensue where future interactions are still plagued by the unresolved issues. Whilst there may be times to put off difficult conversations until the appropriate environment and time can be found (i.e. behind closed doors and definitely not in front of patients), I would encourage you not to let things fester. For those of you whose personalities naturally avoid conflict, it may have to be learned behaviour to seek conflict out in order to resolve it.

The wisest option of all (yes, I have slipped in the clichéd owl option) is for both parties to express their needs clearly and calmly and find a joint solution that manages to fulfil all of those needs. This would be classed as the assertive or win–win approach.

Of course, in reality, victory for one person may automatically have negative consequences for the other. In the complex realm of healthcare it may involve a degree of compromise and cooperation on both sides to achieve something that feels equitable to everyone involved, with some winning and some losing being experienced on both sides but in equal amounts. I thought this might need the intelligence, agility, and sense of humour that the dolphin signifies for me.

Being able to express your needs assertively is vital. To recap, *assertive* is a word that is often used incorrectly when people actually mean aggressive. Assertive actually means that you are expressing your needs or feelings. 'I feel . . .', 'I think . . .'. We can also include the situation, behaviour, impact, and change or continue (SBIC) approach under this umbrella.

If both parties are able to express their needs in a non-confrontational and balanced way, it is then possible to look at the common ground and potentially move towards agreement. Resolution should either result in ending up in the top right-hand box on Figure 4.1 (win–win/owl–owl) or the middle box (compromise, both parties do some winning and some losing/dolphin–dolphin). That sounds easy, so why doesn't it happen (see Example 4.1)?

Example 4.1 A story about conflict; the ostrich/tortoise approach

There was a team that had two consultants who were originally friends. No-one really understood when or what happened but a problem arose between them. It became so serious that the two consultants no longer wished to be in the same room together. None of the team was brave enough to intervene or to suggest that anyone else intervene either. This made meetings about shared patients at the very least challenging, and in reality completely inadequate. The team learned not to mention the name of one consultant to the other, and vice versa. The consultants had to cover for each other's patients when they were on call. The management of the patients changed according to which consultant was 'on'. The team learned that Dr X liked things one way and so it was done that way on those days, and Dr Y liked it differently and so on those days it was changed. No-one was brave enough to challenge the hierarchy or the conflict. The conflict went on for years and was only resolved when one of them retired. It is difficult to defend this situation as patient care could be compromised by this conflict. It should have been resolved. It may well have needed a mediator to help it become so, and we will discuss that role further on in the chapter.

Prevention is better than cure for personalized conflict

As with anything in healthcare prevention is the ideal. It is better to prevent the personalized conflict in the first place than to have to resolve it after an emotional outburst when damage has already be done.

I want to revisit the concept of whom and what presses your buttons and whose buttons do you press.

I want to start with some personality 'rubs' (see Example 4.2).

Example 4.2 Personal examples of extrovert/introvert

I am an extrovert in Myers–Briggs terms. This manifests itself in a number of ways, but one noticeable way is that I have a tendency to think out loud. I am lucky to share an office with someone who has the same Myers–Briggs style as I do. She is tolerant of me sitting there and talking to my computer or talking to myself as I coach myself through a process. She is tolerant because she understands me and because she behaves in the same way. We laugh about it when we catch ourselves doing it.

However, when I co-facilitate with someone who has a strong 'I' (introvert) preference I try very hard to modify my behaviour. As I arrange the chairs for a teaching session and wonder which layout would suit the session best, I would naturally commentate on my decision-making process (a useful habit in a crisis setting but not necessary with chair layouts). When my introverted colleague is trying to focus on preparing handouts and slides, I began to realize that perhaps my commentating might niggle and interrupt his train of thought.

There are other times when my thinking aloud has caused conflict. My memories are of working in a particular eye theatre. I was very junior and the surgeon was extremely eminent. Everyone in his team knew that he liked to work in silence, but I was new to that team. I was passing through a stable team but no-one told me how the team liked to function. My usual chatty, inquisitive approach coupled with my commentating on my decision making resulted in a rather explosive reaction in this setting which has stayed with me, even though it was 20 years ago. I suspect the surgeon had forgotten about it before the end of the list. Of course, this particular conflict could have been avoided with a briefing in the morning. The conversation could have covered when the hot spots occur and when the sterile cockpit should be used. If the needs of the surgeon had been expressed as 'these are the times when I need to concentrate so I like a bit of quiet', the outburst may never have happened. Whilst it may be unpleasant for me to work in that atmosphere, it is potentially rather more serious. We know that post conflict either the surgeon or myself would be more likely to make an error subsequently.

This example covers only one aspect of a personality interaction using only one model. According to the Myers–Briggs classification or type indicator (MBTI), there are 16 personality types. In addition we have the Belbin[1] preferred team roles (nine options), and the Honey and Mumford[2] preferred learning styles (four main preferences but usually a mixture of more than one) (see Level One pp. 64–5). If we were to take a mathematical approach to personality (not something I would advocate) it is possible to start to see why there are so many possible permutations and combinations. Not surprisingly, you can't expect to get along with everyone.

It isn't just aspects of our personalities that may cause a clash. It can be a host of other behaviours, values, perceptions, social interactions, identities, or interpretations.

It may also be our mood. We have already talked about the concept of a 'Mood Hoover': someone who is inherently negative or repeatedly cynical and tends to looks on the pessimistic side of things—'it will never work!', 'we've already tried that!', 'it's always the same!' The non-verbal equivalent might be rolling one's eyes, tutting or huffing or shaking one's head at suggestions. For me there is no place for a pessimist in the health service (Box 4.1).

Box 4.1 Warning—soap-box moment

We are there to care. We are there to try to do our best. We are not there to moan in front of our patients. Our patients should not know that we are tired or over-stretched. We should make each and every one feel like we have the time for him or her, that he or she is an individual whose needs we care about. If you don't aspire to that I would question whether healthcare is for you. I am not asking us to be superhuman but it should be what we aim and strive for!

The Mood Hoover lowers morale and encourages conflict. I long for the day when we recruit for values, not simply for knowledge and skills. I hope these will include optimism. It is on the list for NASA recruits so why not for a person in healthcare?

I would like us to take care with our use of language. We should avoid sweeping generalizations ('so and so *always* ...', 'we *never* have x equipment ready when I need it!'). We should avoid negative phrases ('we will *never* get through this in the time allowed!', 'oh, if we must!', 'it's more exciting watching paint dry').

Here are some of the aspects of behaviour that healthcare staff told us that pushes buttons and causes conflict: emotional triggers, frustration, over-confidence or lack of confidence, lack of motivation or interest, prejudice, aggression, laziness or apathy, inducing fear, dishonesty, rudeness, and snobbery.

Are you guilty of any of those? Or, almost more importantly, could you give the impression that you are so that this might be someone's perception of you, even if you think it is not the case? It is possible that someone might appear, for example, to lack motivation when really they are simply not as effusive as we are.

These negative qualities are not helpful in our team. If they are present then we need to challenge the poor behaviour (consider using SBIC) and not condone it. Whilst we may not be able to change our personalities, we can alter our behaviour.

What behaviours do you exhibit that could be misconstrued? How could you modify those behaviours or explain them more clearly so that they are not misinterpreted? Do you explain your needs to people? Do you run a good briefing session to explain to your team how you want things done and find out about their needs too? Does your team know where the potential 'rubs' or friction points might lie? Have these been discussed? Do you then revisit these and see how it is all going? Do you try to monitor the performance of the team continually and strive to improve it?

Or is you style more akin to the ostrich?

Resolving the conflict: The role of mediation

Let us move on and assume that despite our best efforts at trying to avoid conflict, it has arisen. We have been unable to negotiate either a win–win situation or a compromise and the result is ongoing conflict. Now what do we do?

I want to introduce the conflict triangle at this point (see Figure 4.2).

A mediator may help to uncover the three sides of the conflict triangle; the people (who is fighting and where are the clashes), the process (how does the conflict manifest itself), and the underlying problem (what they are fighting about).

Mediation in a nutshell

A mediator is impartial and is not there to judge or to find solutions. The mediator's role is to facilitate and encourage shared solutions from the participants. Who the mediator is needs to be agreed by both parties in advance. Ground rules need to be set and a neutral venue agreed. The environment in which the meeting is to be held needs to be well planned to create the right atmosphere. There should be bleep-, phone-, and gadget-free time agreed and a genuine commitment made to giving it a go. It is best if both parties wait in a neutral area and can be invited in to the mediation room together.

The first part of the meeting is used to explore the situation, the second part to reach resolution. Prior to this a reiteration of the ground rules should be made, and there should be a settling-in phase in which parties might establish a rapport. A discussion about what mediation is and what it is not should occur. The confidentiality of the mediation needs to be discussed and the how the report will be drafted. Is the mediation seen as voluntary? The structure of the session should be discussed so that parties know what to expect.

The format is usually run as follows: establishing grounds rules and rapport; listening; exchange; topics established; option generation; decision making; agreement and closure.[3]

There are parallels with the coaching model TGROW (topic, goal, reality, options, and wrap up)[4] which we will cover later in this chapter, as well as parallels with the decision-making models that we have already covered (DODAR[5] and DECIDE).

I am going to outline the mediation process briefly before mentioning some of the techniques that might be used. (Of course, there are many types of mediation and what I'm outlining here is a high level overview of one type.)

After the initial settling-in phase (opening)[3] time is allowed for each participant to express his/her views on what the problem is and its background; this is the

PEOPLE

Who is fighting and how are they experiencing it?
- Personalities, mood
- Emotions, hurts, longings
- Empathy, affection
- Values, interpretations
- Behaviours, skills, abilities
- Identities
- Perceptions of self, other
- Patterns of interaction
- Relative social status
- Relationship roles & history, degree of intimacy

PROCESS

How are they fighting?
- How people communicate
- How discussions go
- How information is handled
- Who is included, excluded
- Structures, systems
- Procedures, laws, rules, & enforcement
- Authority, roles
- Division of responsibilities
- Norms about how to behave in a conflict
- How decisions are made

PROBLEM

What are they fighting about?
- Disagreements
- Concerns, worries
- Blame, accusation
- Explanations and reasons
- Positions, proposed solutions
- Fallouts from past
- Information, data, facts
- Interests, needs, wants
- Interdependence of parties
- Limits, systems, laws, rules
- Subject-matter specifics, technicalities
- Perceived options and consequences

Figure 4.2 The conflict triangle.

Reproduced with permission from Beer, JEB, Packard, CC, and Stief, E, 2012, *The Mediator's Handbook*, 4th edition, Gabriola Island, BC, Canada: New Society Publishers. Copyright © 2012 New Society Publishers.

listening[3] phase. Participants should be listened to without interruption, with the other party taking notes if they wish to. The other party then has his/her turn to speak. This listening phase should be facilitated carefully and is designed to get the problems aired.

The next phase is the ***exchange***.[3] In this phase there is a chance to explore things now that all parties have been heard. This is the time to consider how the behaviours raised affect each other and is best backed up with examples. It can be a time to revisit any notes made and to fill in any gaps, and check that everything is out in the open. We are still at the stage of defining the problems; we are not ready for solutions yet.

Once everyone agrees that all relevant aspects of the problem have been aired, the next stage involves generating the ***topic list***.[3] This is a summary of all of the problems, grouped together in themes so that the overall number of topics does not exceed about five (returning to the seven plus or minus two theme from earlier).[6]

Once the topic list is generated we move to the ***option generation***[3] phase. This can initially be a bit like a brainstorming session where no idea is discarded. Every topic raised needs to be covered. The mediator doesn't sit in judgement on the solutions but instead encourages as many as possible to be considered.

The next stage is the ***decision-making***[3] phase where the solution for each topic is selected. For me there are again very strong parallels with coaching, educational supervision, and developmental goals in their various guises. The proposed solutions need to pass a reality test and also need to have full support from both parties. Each decision needs to be specific, achievable, realistic, and possibly have a time scale (this parallels SMART (specific, measurable, achievable, realistic, and timely) goals but perhaps without the measureable component).

Once both parties are happy with the outputs these decisions are documented in an ***agreement***.[3] It is not legally binding. It is worth revisiting the grounds rules here with regards to who can keep a copy of the report and what if anything may be shared/made public outside of the confines of the meeting.

The meeting is brought to an end by reviewing the written agreement and a ***closure***[3] phase.

Mediation is not a magic wand. It is not up to the mediator to find solutions; it is the interested parties who must find solutions with the mediator helping them do so. It can take more than one meeting to complete the process.

Batman, mediator, and coaching tools

I alluded to Batman in Level One (p. 69; pp. 148–9). If you think of yourself as a superhero (tights and underpants on the outside entirely optional!) you would have an all-important utility belt. In the utility belt are a range of techniques and skills. Not only do you need to understand the tools and to have practised with them, you also need to ensure that you choose the right one (or combination of them) to use at the right time.

I want to introduce some of the techniques that mediators and coaches use as I suspect they could be useful in any team. These tools can be used in different settings including coaching, debriefing, facilitating, and leadership forums, not just in conflict resolution. In a number of frameworks involving non-technical skills, conflict resolution simply refers to 'resolving conflict', but it doesn't really go into any depth about how to achieve that. What should we actually do or say? What should we avoid doing or saying?

Which tool we can use and when depends on where we are, how many other people are around, whether we are in the middle of an emergency or an urgent clinical situation, the time available, the emotional state of those involved, how well you know them, the hierarchy of those involved, and how experienced you are at handling that sort of conflict.

Let us start with a situation where you are witnessing conflict rather than personally being in the firing line or feeling conflicted.

First do no harm

One of things to *avoid* is to tell someone to 'calm down'. This is simply likely to pour petrol on the fire. Let them vent but listen actively while they do so. You need to listen very hard because in a minute you may need to repeat back some of what they have just said.

Another thing to *avoid* is to tell someone that you 'know how they feel'. You don't know how they feel, you are not them, and even if you have been through something similar you will have experienced it with from your own perspective, from your different background, different value set, different personality, different past experience, and so on. Do not start to regale a similar event that has happened to you. It is time for you to listen and show empathy. And of course, it is important that we show empathy, and there are many effective ways of doing so.

'That sounds like you have a lot on your plate!'

'You seem to be collecting life events; how are you coping with all of that at once?'

'That sounds tough!'

If we consider conflict in its most basic form as someone feeling that his or her needs are not being met, it is a good starting point to establish what those needs might be.

121

Listening and the use of silence

Perhaps the most important skill of all when confronted by a conflict situation is listening. I find when teaching this as a skill that some members of the healthcare community are slightly arrogant about this. We seem to assume that because we should be caring, empathic, and good listeners that naturally we are just this. I too was guilty of the *assumption* that my listening skills weren't bad until I went on my coaching course. I had my listening skills unpicked for a whole day before they were re-assembled and honed.

I am going to break listening into steps.

Non-verbal

Facial expression

I want you to imagine that it is Christmas and we playing charades again but ideally you are going to watch yourself in a mirror instead. I want you to imagine that your charade is '*interested*'. Looking at yourself in the mirror. I want you to perfect your 'interested' face. Someone in a conflict setting needs to know that you are really listening, but we should be looking interested in what our patients are saying, or interested in what their relatives are able to add, or interested in what another member of staff is saying. Looking interested is harder than it sounds. Looking interested yet natural, with an uncontorted face is even harder.

Eye contact

Achieving the correct amount of eye contact can be tricky. We do not want the person we are working with to feel like we are fixing them with a hard stare, but we do want to be paying attention and listening actively. Don't worry if the person you are working with looks away from you; people often break eye contact when they are thinking. We are generating a thinking partnership and this is a positive sign.

Stillness

If you are talking and thinking it can be very distracting to have the person in front of you fidgeting or doing something distracting. Try to become aware of whether your body is moving or still. The best way to find out about whether you are guilty of this is to ask for feedback at the end of a session or, if you can bear it, to be filmed while you are listening.

Posture

I am not a believer in adopting a certain posture while you are listening. I know that traditionally some communication skills courses taught a 'lean in, head tilt, touch knee' approach. I hope they have moved on.

You should understand the difference between an open and a closed posture. Leaning in a little but not too much can be helpful. Not looking so casual that it seems as if you are not engaged should be balanced with looking relaxed and not too formal. Natural mirroring (adopting the posture of the person opposite you) is supposed to help people feel more comfortable but don't overdo it.

Attention

You will need to be really paying attention to what the person is saying. This means that you need to be able to clear your thoughts from all of the distractions of your day. How are you going to do that?

Once you have cleared your head of your own distractions (this is sometimes referred to as being 'present'), you then have to stay aware throughout the whole episode. It is important that you consciously steer away from letting similar experiences creep into your mind. It is equally important that you don't jump ahead and start thinking of solutions.

If you think this is something you would like to explore in more depth, I have found the technique of mindfulness very helpful with this.

Even if you don't buy into the whole idea of doing mindfulness training, at the very least take five minutes before the consultation/session to catch your breath and clear your thoughts. You need to move from whatever you were doing (probably rushing around under high workload and time pressure) and change into 'still, calm, interested, listening mode'.

It is vital that the person feels that you have time to listen. So if you do have a time constraint mention that at the beginning of the session, apologize for it, and consider offering a follow-up time when you have no pressure. Better still would be to delegate the other task so that you can give someone your full attention.

Periodically you can do a balcony and a dance floor[7] micro-check. Just sneak up to the balcony and look at yourself on the dance floor. How am I doing with my attention here? To listen while you do this takes practice.

A surprising number of people are uncomfortable with silence. People that have yet to master the use of silence fall into the pitfalls of trying to fill the conversational gaps with either another question or a summary or a statement. In fact, if the person can't answer your question straight away, you can reward yourself as you have probably asked a good, probing question that has encouraged thinking. In either coaching or a conflict setting I would advise you to just sit tight and wait and allow time for people to think.

If we move away from conflict resolution for a second and think of other times when you can practise these skills. I want you to imagine a more educational setting. If you are facilitating or debriefing a group and you reach a silence, initially the same advice applies; just wait. Have a look around the group to see if the floor suddenly looks very interesting as everyone is trying to avoid your gaze. Try signalling non-verbally either with some brief eye contact or an open palm or a slight beckoning action. Depending on the topic, if you have waited as long as you seem able, consider whether it might be appropriate to name what you are observing. 'I can see that the floor is very interesting right now and you are all avoiding my gaze. I wonder why that might be?' You have to use your judgement here. Is there a dynamic in the room that makes the topic tricky? Have you lost your audience? Is there an elephant in the room that no-one is brave enough to name? Is there a knowledge gap that no-one wants to admit to, or is your audience tired and in need of a break? Are they deep in thought and find that you are rushing them? Have you exhausted the topic and they have run out of ideas? Are they feeling stressed by who else is in the room and so can't think clearly? Are they afraid of stating the obvious and looking daft?

A couple of the last options lead me to talk about making a session psychologically and physically safe.

Safety

We need to make sure that in a potential conflict setting we are safe. You need a plan of what you might do if things got heated. You need to decide where the meeting will be, who might be nearby, and how you might extricate yourself if need be. You need to consider who should be present with you. If you suspect this might be an issue, you need to introduce at the outset the possibility of calling for a pause in proceedings. In an ideal setting you would know whether there is any history of angry outbursts from the party concerned and if so whether any of these has resulted in violence.

Building a rapport between yourself and another individual or a group is essential for resolving conflict, coaching, facilitating, and debriefing. The approach differs depending on which of these four activities are undertaken.

◆ For facilitating, I use a series of 'ice-breakers' and I don't go past these until I feel that the group has warmed up and all given something.

◆ Debriefing: I will cover later in the book.

◆ Coaching: I spend at least half an hour of the first meeting establishing ground rules and settling in before we actually start the coaching session. (This is known as contracting, something you may periodically repeat throughout a session.)

◆ Conflict resolution. It is important that if you are meeting with two parties everything seems fair to both. As with coaching the first phase sets what to expect, what mediation is and is not, and lets the parties become comfortable with what lies ahead.

Don't move beyond the first stage if you don't feel you have established a rapport with them. It can be helpful to introduce the concept of 'challenge'; ask what the person feels this might mean, discuss how the level of challenge might be able to increase with an increasing level of rapport, and why this might be useful.

It is important to build an atmosphere of psychological safety in all the settings.

This involves the parties feeling that they won't be judged and so they can be honest and say what they really think. In a learning setting, it means generating an atmosphere of 'it's OK to have a go'.

There is an element of trust that we need to build. There may be an element of credibility required within generating this trust. 'You seem to know what you are doing so I'm willing to have a go at this process!'

Layout of the room

Think about *where* you are so that other people, or phones, or bleeps won't interrupt the conversation. It needs to be somewhere neutral where the person feels relaxed and able to think. You need to plan the room's layout so that it is comfortable, without information displayed that will distract attention away from the matter at hand. Chairs should be comfortable, an appropriate distance apart, and angled so that it does not appear as if an interview or a confrontation is about to take place, but so that you can still maintain eye contact when required.

Use of language

We need to be able to use 'clean' language that isn't open to misinterpretation and is not ambiguous. (There is a television advert that I use as a metaphor for this: it passes the Ronseal® test and 'it does what it says on the tin'.)

There is also something about being able to dig a bit deeper under the surface. When the person uses a word or phrase, maintain your curiosity about what meaning they intended to convey rather than making an assumption that you already have a shared understanding. 'Can you clarify that a little for me please?' 'Tell me more about that.'

Learning to use appropriate metaphors and understand their meaning is also a useful skill to grasp.

Open questions

We mentioned open questions in Level One. We are going to revisit this as our first technique.

When I run training sessions on this people can usually tell me that a closed question can be answered with a 'yes' or 'no' answer. There is also the semi-closed question that can be answered with a one-word answer other than 'yes' or 'no'; for example 'whose idea was it?' Despite the fact that most people know what a closed question is they find it difficult not to fall into the trap of using one.

If we want someone to talk to us and explain how and why he or she is experiencing conflict, we want to do this without asking leading questions or making assumptions. Closed questions are sometimes used because the person asking them has already found a solution to the problem in their head and now they want to lead the individual towards this answer.

I do not want you to have an answer. If it is not your conflict, it is not your role to find the solution. A better solution will be found and agreed by those involved in the conflict. Your role is to help them find their own solution, and this may or may not be possible.

The first step is to help them express to each other or to you what the issues are. This is best achieved with open questions.

When people are learning this technique, they often struggle. My first tip is to start your sentences with 'how'.

'How did that come about?'

'How was that decision made?'

'How did that experience affect you?'

'How has it been working together?'

'How did that manifest itself?'

Once you have mastered the 'how' move on to trying 'what?'

'What was going through your mind at that point?'

'What happened next?'

'What else?'

Then you try mixing them together. After you have mastered this you can practice adding in other questions. Who? When? Where? (But don't ask 'why'. 'Why' can be perceived as a more aggressive approach. See below.) It takes practice to become good at questioning; just knowing the theory is not enough. Like any skill, you will not master it instantly.

The seven tests for a question*

1. What is my *intent*?

2. What will the *impact* of my question be?

3. Is it the right *time* to ask it?

4. Is the *relationship* ready? (Have I built up enough trust and rapport?)

5. Will it raise *awareness*?

6. Will it leave *responsibility for the solution with the participants*?

7. Will it leave *choice with the participants*?

   With regard to both of the last questions, try to make sure that you are not coming up with solutions for the participants nor trying to close down the options for which solutions they may wish to consider.

*Adapted from The Performance Coach (2011). *ILM Level 7 Certificated Coaching Programme* (Resource Guide prepared by The Performance Coach for NHS South Central). Copyright © 2011 The Performance Coach, Ltd.

We are trying to leave responsibility for the problem solving with those with the problem. We are there to shift perceptions and encourage thinking. We don't have to have the answers ourselves.

You have to believe in the people you are working with. You have to trust that they can solve problems themselves. In fact, they will find a better solution than you can because they know all the facts and the context better than you do. They are in the best place to find a solution that will work.

I remember being overwhelmed by the seven questions when I was first learning to coach. I was under the impression that I simultaneously had to ask myself the seven questions about each question I was asking someone else. Of course, that would be impossible. A good technique is to nip up to the balcony now and again and peek at yourself asking the question and consider just one of the seven questions.

My tip would be to start to focus on responsibility. Am I leaving responsibility for the solution with the person/people I'm working with?

After you have mastered question 6, then try some of the others. Remember that being timely is important; it may have been a good question earlier in a conversation but if you miss the moment you can interrupt the person's thought processes.

Prompts

The questions can be interspersed with prompts.

'Tell me more about that.'

'What happened next?'

'And then?'

'Can you expand on that?'

'What else?'

Avoid the question 'why?'

In both mediation and coaching we are encouraged either to avoid or at the very least be cautious with any question beginning with the word 'why?' Experts have found that this word can be too confrontational and too direct. If you find yourself being inquisitive about why something happened, check with yourself first. Do you really need to know? Will the answer benefit the person you are trying to help?

If you think it is important then either soften it with a 'how' question or use a prompt instead.

'How did you decide to take that course of action?'

'Tell me more about that decision.'

Clarifying questions and information gathering

Of course, we are not banning closed questions completely but bear in mind the ratio of open to closed question. It can be useful to narrow down a time scale ('when will you achieve that by?'), or make sure there is clear role allocation ('who will be handling that?'). These kinds of questions come under the heading of zooming in. (Imagine you are in the broad bit of the funnel that we mentioned in Level One and that you are moving toward the detail.)

It can also be useful in some settings to reverse this and zoom out: 'how would you put that in the context of the department/organization?'

It may be that you just don't understand what they are trying to say. If this is the case, it is best that you take responsibility for not understanding rather than inferring that they are the ones who are failing to make any sense.

'Let me just pause there for a second and recap. What I've heard so far is … but I'm not sure I fully grasped the next bit. Can you just go over that part again for me?'

'Help me understand …'.

It is important to unpick 'assumptions' which can also be known as 'mind reads'. This is, as the name suggests, when one party has made an assumption about what someone else was thinking or intending.

'I can hear your take on that; let's just explore what Jeremy meant by … '.

There may be ambiguity that needs to be clarified.

Remember when you are gathering a list of problems that the order in which they are presented does not relate to the order of their importance. Once you have already gathered some information and you want to check whether it is complete or whether there are more issues to be covered, use the word 'something' rather than the word 'anything'. For example, 'was there something else?'

It is worth challenging sweeping generalizations such as 'she always ...', or 'he never ...', or 'every single time we ...'.

A useful challenge might be 'are there times when it happens differently?'

Hypothesis testing

This has two parts. This involves making a statement first (usually an observation). Then we ask a question to see how the hypothesis has 'landed'.

'I noticed when you were talking about ... that you seemed ... I wondered what are your thoughts about that?'

This can help to highlight feelings and perceptions that you think might be useful to name or to encourage insight.

Appreciative enquiry

There is a growing emphasis in putting a positive spin on a question. This fits in with the glass-half-full approach that I like. It also fits in with an approach where people play to their strengths rather than work on their weaknesses which tends to make them focus on what they can't do.

It can be useful to encourage the parties to find a similar situation when they have used the skills they might need to solve this problem? You could highlight the fact that the skills they need already exist, and ask whether or not they can then adapt them to the new setting.

With this approach, the questions focus on what is working well, and the amplification of these. Lessons are then drawn from what has worked rather than from problems or mistakes.

Summarizing / paraphrasing / reflecting back / pre-framing

Another key tool in the mediator's toolbox is the power of the summary. In fact, Whatling[8] describes summarizing as the 'Swiss Army knife' in the mediator's toolbox.

Put simply you are going to summarize what someone has said.

Let's break down the basic idea of summarizing into component parts: you have to listen like mad, remember what has been said, process and filter the information to pick out the key points without missing any of the vital parts but simultaneously removing the unnecessary bits, also remove all the emotive words that may cause a negative reaction in the other person, and repeat it back in a balanced non-judgemental tone that is engaging and impartial. Now it doesn't sound quite so easy.

Summarizing can be used effectively with an individual in a coaching session, in a group debrief, in a shuttle mediation when you are seeing one party and then the other, or in a mediation where both parties are present.

It achieves a number of different aims. Here are ten examples:

◆ It shows that you are listening and giving the individual your attention. When you are in a conflict situation you may need to feel heard, you may need to feel that someone is 'finally' taking your concerns seriously.

◆ It demonstrates an understanding by the mediator of what is going on.

◆ It offers an opportunity for clarification and redirection by the party if he or she feels the mediator hasn't quite got it right.

◆ It can have an interesting effect hearing your thoughts spoken out loud when previously they represent only an internal dialogue. It can shift perceptions.

◆ It can help filter and get to the nub of problem that could be hidden within lots of facts or clouded by emotion.

◆ Summarizing can be used to try to redirect attention or to highlight something that may not currently being given enough thought.

◆ It can be used when things seem a bit stuck.

◆ It can be used to signal that we think we are ready to move to the next step of the process and to check that both parties are also ready to move on.

◆ It can be used to check that we have gathered all of the information. 'This is what we have so far … '. 'Was there something else?'

◆ It is used as part of closure.

Pre-framing and paraphrasing

It can be important for micro-summaries that we make it clear whether we are going to use our own words or those of the party we are trying to help. To try and maintain the rapport of the person we are working with it can help to make this clear when you are summarizing. We do this by 'pre-framing' what we are going to say.

'What I think I heard was …'.

'Using my words, what I have learned so far is … '.

The 'paraphrasing' is when we use our words rather than the words of the person involved in the conflict. This can be used to soften what was originally said and reframe it so that it is less likely to evoke a negative emotion in the second party.

It is also harder to remember words verbatim and rather than get it wrong, it can be better to summarize the understanding of the words and make sure you have that right, rather than to place too much emphasis on the exact wording itself.

I would like you to practise this skill. For this you will need a willing friend/spouse/team-mate, or even better, persuade two people to do the following with you. When you have found someone, I would like him or her to start reading Exercise 4.1. You must not peek at the example (how tempted are you?), and you must only listen to the instructions they give you.

Exercise 4.1 Practice example for listening and summary skills

Instructions for your helper—no peeking

Do not read this bit aloud. Thanks for agreeing to help with this. In a few lines I'm going to ask you to read aloud the passage that is in italics. The aim is to help with listening and summarizing skills.

You will need to pretend to be two different people who are having a disagreement, or if there are two of you, take a role each. I would like you to choose two characters from a list depending on who you think would be most appropriate for the person you are practising with (from now on I will refer to this person as the 'listener').

Two nurses, and the listener is the sister-in-charge.

Two midwives, and the listener is the midwife who draws up the rota.

Two doctors, and the listener is the rota lead.

Two other healthcare professionals who work shifts on a rota, and the listener draws up the rota.

It might be useful to have pen and paper handy.

Please share the roles you have chosen with your listener and give each character a name. Inform the listener that the task is to listen to two people and then summarize the key points from each viewpoint. At the end of person 1's speech, please can you summarize the key points made. At the end of person 2's speech, please summarize.

I am going to ask you to read two passages out loud. At the end of the first passage I want you to wait and allow the listener to summarize all of the key points. Then please read person 2 aloud. The listener then needs to summarize the key points from person 2.

Please read aloud what is written in italics:

I am going to start with ... ... (person 1). I will then pause and wait for you to summarize. When ... ... (person 2) has finished you must summarize what has been said. We will then review your summaries. Are you happy that you understand the instructions?

If they are happy, proceed. If not, please repeat the last section.

Person 1

I am completely fed up. I've got Christmas day and New Year's Eve and I worked Christmas Day last year. (Person 2) hasn't done any bank holidays. They have had all the holidays and breaks that they have asked for and I never get what I ask for. We are trying to have a big family party this year. I've got my sister coming from France and my Mum is coming to stay. We haven't had the family all together for over three years since my Dad died. I'm really not seeing enough of my children, it's causing terrible problems at home. I've really had enough!

Stop talking. Wait and allow the listener to summarize. Try to see if he/she remembers all of the points you have just read out. Write down any that he/she misses.

Person 2

You can't play the children card. Just because I don't have children doesn't mean that I should work Christmas. I have already swapped my week of nights with you last month to try to help you out and now here you are moaning! I've been doing an exam so I had to have some time off to do that. I want to go skiing at Christmas and so I requested that time off months ago. You think you are more important because you have a family; well I have a life too! Why should your family be more important than my life?

Wait and allow the listener to summarize. Listen to see if he/she included all of the facts. Write down any that have been missed.

How did they do? How did it feel to be listened to? Does the listener have any distracting habits? Did the listener look interested in what you were saying? Were the summaries accurate? Do you think the summary would have helped to calm things down a bit or would it have inflamed things? Please explain your thoughts to your listener and give them some feedback.

Some other common pitfalls when people are learning this technique are included next.

Avoid the double question

What I commonly observe is that people start with an open question but it doesn't quite come out in the way that they intended. They tend to ask it again but phrase it slightly differently without having allowed the first version to be answered. This is one version of what I call the 'double question'. The person trying to answer the question becomes confused about which version of the question they are now supposed to be answering and it distracts them from thinking, which is what we want them to be doing.

It doesn't matter if your question isn't perfect; no-one else knew what you were trying to ask anyway. Just see what it elicits. You can always redirect afterwards.

The second type of 'double question' that I observe is one where people are uncomfortable with silence. It can be that they have asked a great question.

(You can tell that you've asked a great question when someone has to take time to think before they answer. Incidentally, it is worth getting to know what someone's 'thinking face' is like when you are working with them in this sort of setting. No two people have the same thinking face; it is a very individual thing. As already discussed, I often find that they break eye contact for a bit while they think.)

After the great question comes the silence and the thinking. The questioner, uncomfortable with this silence, feels the need to fill it, and does so by asking either another question or a different version of the same question.

Be brave, sit tight, and just wait.

The third type of 'double question' is something that just becomes too complicated and has multiple parts to it and is best simply asked one part at a time. This fits with the next principle.

Keep it short and sweet

Another common pitfall is to overcomplicate the question. By shortening it up, it often broadens out the question, allowing more thinking and a greater depth for the answer.

Other coaching competencies that will help in a conflict setting

There are 12 coaching competencies; I am only including three of those here.

Self-awareness

This encompasses some of what we referred to earlier as being aware of where your attention is directed. In coaching it is referred to as being 'present'. This means that you have emptied your bucket before the session begins. You are not thinking about any of your personal stresses, or what happened to you as you travelled in that morning, or your meeting later in the day. You clear your mind of any interference. It also means that you are aware of any emotions or responses or triggers in you that occur during the session. You are aware of the impact your body language, your facial expression, your words, and your tone of voice have on the session and on the people with whom you are working.

I recommend developing mindfulness to help you master this skill.

Self-management

Self-management is the next step after you realize an emotional response has been triggered in you during the session. You have to have sufficient emotional intelligence not only to be able to understand but also to effectively manage your personal opinions, views, and attitudes. You need to be able to switch off your personal judgement about either of the individuals whom you are trying to help.

Beliefs and attitudes

This is about *really* believing in the potential of the people you are working with. If you go into a session believing that there will be a successful outcome to the session, the people in the room will pick up this feeling.

It is important that you understand that when two people recall something from an event they may have completely different accounts. This does not mean that one of them is lying; they are just interpreting things from their own perspectives, value sets, life experiences, and memory recall.

It is important to demonstrate empathy across the wide realms of cultural diversity.

More advanced techniques for resolving conflict

'Normalizing'

When both parties believe that their conflict is unique and unsolvable, the harder it will be to bring them back to common ground. Once you have established a rapport and gained the trust of both parties, this technique involves acknowledging that conflict is not unusual. It acknowledges that considering the situation they are in, it is perhaps not surprising that conflict has arisen. This is combined with a sense of balanced optimism that there will be ways to resolve the conflict.

People will have resolved conflict before this one occurred. We are going to help them believe that they can solve this one too, but we can't solve it for them. It can be worth pointing out that sometimes conflict is a necessary part of change, but be careful not to sound too preachy or parental!

'Mutualizing'

If we are going to succeed we will need to shift perceptions of what is right and wrong and may have to help alter entrenched viewpoints.

One of the ways we might subtly unpick some of the 'certainty' that each party initially has that 'they are right', can involve a technique called 'mutualization'.

For example, the mediator may emphasize that what he or she has heard is that the parties are poles apart in their descriptions of what has happened up until this point, but there seems to be lots of common ground about wanting to work together to give the best possible care to patients.

Past-to-future state

In the example above, I have also encompassed a little of this technique too. I have referred to people being poles apart in the past but implied positivity about the future way of working together. If the conflict keeps returning to what has happened in the past, it is important to try to bring it back to moving forwards or redirecting to the future. (It may also be important, however, to identify where the problem is and which need has not yet been met.)

Concatenation

This is really a fancy term for combining some of the techniques we have been discussing.

Positive reframing

This one is more challenging and needs to be practised. It has similarities to summarizing but instead of just repeating what you have heard, you:

1. filter it,

2. process it, and

3. repackage it.

During the filtering phase, you remove emotions, judgements, inflammatory remarks, and assumptions. This all happens in your head rather than out loud.

In the processing phase, you either pick out just the facts or perhaps in a more complicated scenario, the unmet need. This all happens in your head too.

You then rephrase things with a positive spin and deliver this aloud. Try this out with the examples in Exercise 4.2.

Exercise 4.2 Have a go at positive reframing

Grab a paper and a pen and see if you can write down what you might say to produce positive reframing of the following.

1. I am fed up with the way you roll your eyes and tut at me!

2. You keep leaving early! I've had enough! Why should I cover your patients when you've gone just because you are part time?

3. I don't understand why you keep sending me all of these aggressive emails!

4. You keep undermining me in front of the junior members of staff!

Even if you haven't written them down, try and have a go at each one before you go read on.

Sample reframing:

1. I am wondering whether when one of you is cross—would you like to be more up front about things and have a conversation about it?

2. It sounds like there is a high workload on your ward. What I'm hearing is that you would like clearer rules about what happens with patients when staff have differing shift times, have I got that right?

3. What I'm picking up is, when there is an issue, you would like to talk together as the emotion in emails can be easily misinterpreted. How does that sound?

4. What I think I'm hearing is, when there is an issue to be discussed, you would like that conversation to take place in a suitable place behind closed doors where it can't be overheard by more junior staff.

They are all phrased as questions or with an element of uncertainty, so that if you haven't got it quite right then the parties have another chance to say what they intended to mean.

Hierarchy and its influence in conflict

We have mentioned repeatedly the importance of the hierarchy and how if it is too steep it can inhibit patient safety. I want to revisit this notion here in the context of conflict. Remembering that conflict can take many forms; it may be that a steep hierarchy inhibits people from expressing their needs or their concerns.

A few '*thought bubbles*' to ponder:

'If only they weren't so scary, I might say something.'

'I'm sure they must know what they are doing, they are a consultant/matron/very senior/very experienced.'

'I really feel like I should do something but I don't know how to go about it.'

'They must have seen *it* (it being the allergy band or the bleeding vessel or the fact that the side is wrong or the blood pressure has dropped or the patient is unconscious, etc.). Maybe I am missing something? I wonder if I should say something?'

In these examples, the more junior team member feels unable to express him or herself when he or she witnesses something that the other individual does not see as a problem. The conflicting views haven't surfaced. The conflict is undeclared and the team continues down a potentially incorrect path with an error looming on the horizon.

We have, I hope, already emphasized the importance of a leader inviting ideas from his or her team and flattening that hierarchy by making him or herself appear to be more approachable.

I now want to add an extra tool for assertiveness that the team members can use to challenge when something might be going wrong. The very firm message is 'yes, please say something'. Please speak up, and if someone has spoken up, listen to him or her and treat the idea raised respectfully, no matter what his or her grade. Everyone should have a voice. Anyone can make a mistake and anyone can spot one.

Assertiveness

There is a mnemonic teams can use to learn to express what is known as graded assertiveness. It is a pre-agreed framework with a number of trigger words that should help both the person trying to be assertive but also be recognizable by those on the team who are listening to the verbal cues.

Graded assertiveness

The mnemonic is CUSS, which stands for Concern, Unsure, Safety, and Stop. The idea is to include each word in a sentence in turn, if required. You continue to escalate to the next sentence until someone listens to you (see Box 4.2).

> # Box 4.2 CUSS
>
> C—CONCERN: I am *concerned* about this patient's penicillin allergy.
>
> U—UNSURE: I am *unsure* that tazocin can be given to someone with a penicillin allergy.
>
> S—SAFETY: I am worried that it's *unsafe* to give this patient tazocin as he has a known allergy to penicillin.
>
> S—STOP: Please *stop.* We need to take a moment while I look it up.

What next?

If we assume that we have managed to resolve the current conflict within a team, the question now arises regarding where do we go next? How do we move things forward so that some of these issues do not simply reappear?

My thoughts are that a 'fiery' conflict between two or more members of a team will have had a very bruising effect. It will be difficult to simply put all of that behind you and move on. My suggestions are that there is a real role for some team coaching or development to build on the successful resolution. Some of the individuals within the team may also benefit from some individual coaching sessions.

Post-conflict team development

I believe it is useful for anyone in a leadership role to have some basic coaching skills. If we think back to Daniel Goleman's[9] work that we explored in Level One, a coaching style of leadership was found to have a very positive effect on the team and on achieving the desired task. Unlike the pacesetting approach, it means that the team will feel empowered to make decisions themselves and will learn far more effectively and the result will be a sustained change, rather than one that is dependent on the micro-management of the leader.

There are many kinds of coaching courses, ranging from a couple of days to a full post-graduate diploma. What I include here is only a taster to whet your appetite for some of the techniques a coach might have to offer. I hope that it will encourage you to attend some more formal training. The NHS is developing a network of coaches and I would suggest using a fully-fledged coach.

So what is coaching?

The easiest way to imagine coaching is as a *'thinking partnership'*.

The image that is commonly used is that the coachee has a tree. The coach is invited to climb up into the tree and sit with the coachee on the same branch of the tree. They can then see the world from the same perspective as the coachee sees it.

When might coaching help?

Coaching is particularly useful during periods of change including when you receive a promotion, or are changing role, or changing job, or have a big life event. It may be that there is a personal relationship either at work or home that is challenging, or you think you might want to develop some new skills (leadership, assertiveness, team working), or there may be a problem on which you feel 'stuck'. All of these settings would be suitable coaching topics.

Coaching is usually a short-term intervention, often between only four and six sessions which help you to achieve the transition, overcome the challenges in the relationship, develop the new skill, or the solve the problem at hand.

Coaching an individual

The most commonly used model for coaching is the GROW model[4] which has been adapted to TGROW. This is the process that forms the basis for the clinical consultation. The coach (hopefully skilfully and almost invisibly) takes responsibility for the process, leaving the responsibility for the content of the session with the coachee. The TGROW model is the framework on which the session sits.

The process is not sequential but switches backwards and forwards between the elements. Within a session all elements are covered.

1. Topic
The first part of the process involves gaining an initial understanding. It is when we start to build rapport and begin to explore what is going on for our coachee. At this point it is a broad overview to build a context for the overall issues.

2. Goal
This is something more specific; what should be the focus of this session? What would success look like at the end of the session?

3. Reality
In this section, things are explored in more detail. It covers the 'who, what, how, how much, and where' of the situation and perhaps also of the solutions they are exploring. The plan is to encourage increased awareness of the situation for the coachee and perhaps a shift in perspective.

4. Options

Much as we have discussed option generation in the decision-making chapter, here to we encourage the coachee to explore multiple ways of achieving the goal he or she has set him/herself.

5. Wrap up / finding the will

In the final stages of the session, it is important to try and firm up what actions the coachee will be taking and how he or she takes the very first steps. The steps of the process need to be very clear but they should have been designed and developed by the coachee as he or she is the person that can find the best solution to meet his or her individual needs. You also need to establish the *will* for them to do it.

Another model

Hawkins[10] suggested another model: CLEAR. Contract, Listen, Explore, Action, and Review. We will return to this in the team section.

Managing the process

Whilst the coach manages the process, the material that is discussed or the content of the session is chosen by the coachee. The framework, TGROW, is simply that: something on which to hang the session. There are then a range of techniques, approaches, and tools that can be used and introduced during the session.

Coaching can include a spectrum of techniques. This spans from working with a very non-directive approach that overlaps with a counselling-type style, to the more directive end of the spectrum where the coach gives advice, overlapping with mentoring. Think of a session being like a tango, and the coach tango dancing along the line of techniques, matching the right technique to the right moment. (I am still happy with my superhero and my utility belt. I think Batman doing a tango maybe taking the metaphor a step too far!) See Figure 4.3 for the range of coaching techniques. This spectrum can also be thought of in terms of 'push–pull': pushing solves someone's problems for them, and pulling encourages them to solve their own problems.

As well as using the range of techniques the coach may introduce a model. Examples of models (think of the tools in your utility belt) include: wisdom with hindsight, appreciative enquiry, the inner game, the change cycle, the leadership pipeline, creative mentoring, components of sustained performance, emotional intelligence, resilience, mind mapping, and organizational systems. There are many more[4,10].

Whilst it may be helpful for one member of the team to have some coaching, a whole-team approach following conflict may be more beneficial.

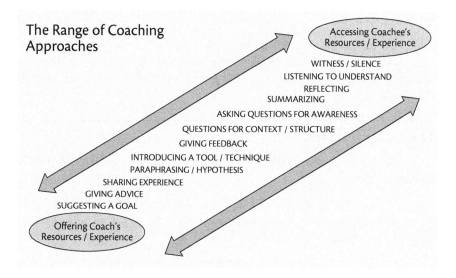

Figure 4.3 The range of coaching approaches.

Reproduced with permission from The Performance Coach (2011). *ILM Level 7 Certificated Coaching Programme* (Resource Guide prepared by The Performance Coach for NHS South Central). Copyright © 2011 The Performance Coach, Ltd (with special thanks to Chris Sheepshanks for his tango-dancing metaphor).

Team development

The starting point may be establishing what the concept of 'team' actually means to the group of people.

Within the team it is important to understand the needs of each individual.

Once we have established what a team is and agreed to engage in building one, the team needs some ground rules for how members will work together and how they will behave. They also need to cover what behaviours might not be acceptable and how to deal with those behaviours, should they occur.

They need to establish how they will make shared decisions.

They then need to put some of this into practice by agreeing the team objectives and how to prioritize those.

Within the team, the roles and functions required to fulfil the agreed team objectives need to be established. Clear responsibility for each role and function must be established too. Ideally this will be achieved in a way that plays to the strengths and interests of the individuals (consider a tool such as Belbin).[1]

The team needs to agree what success will look like and how it will check on its progress.

Who might help?

There are various options for team development including team facilitation, team coaching, and team training. It may be that you have access to someone in a learning and development role who can help with this, or you may need to look further afield.

Team coaching model

It is possible to use the TGROW model for team coaching too but other approaches exist.

Hawkins[10] uses the CLEAR model for team coaching. He focuses on four areas for the coaching and developmental process. What follows is my interpretation of those four areas.

1. External fit—where does this team fit within the organization? In the case of the executive team—where does the organization fit into its external environment? What is the purpose of this team? What is it commissioned to do and by whom?

2. Internal focus—how is the team going to translate that overall purpose and convert it into actions? What other actions might it also need to achieve?

3. How?—how will the team work together? Who will have which roles and responsibilities? What will the team culture be like?

4. Who might the team have to interact with? How will it go about that interaction? What would this look like if it was successful?

I am going to go through this using an example of a group of consultant colorectal surgeons in Example 4.3.

Example 4.3 A team of colorectal surgeons

1) If we start with the external fit, we have a group of individuals from the same profession who should be working together collaboratively. The amount of services that they should be delivering is decided by a negotiation between the local commissioning group and the hospital. In an ideal world (indulge my fantasy) there will be a set number of procedures agreed that will be performed on an agreed number of patients at an agreed tariff that perfectly matches the needs of the local population. This quantity of procedures will have had clinical input and operational input in setting it up so that it is both appropriate and realistic. The team of surgeons will know the content

of the contract, have been party to its agreement, and understand the line-management structure between them and the decision.

How well are the clinical and operational team working together? How is the line management working? How are the processes working? How is the joint decision making working? Is there a shared mental model of how the team members work together? If this team is successful, how will it benefit the patients and the organization?

2) Within the team (i.e. the internal focus), does everyone have a shared understanding of his or her purpose? This might involve understanding how many clinics, how many theatre lists, how many MDTs (multidisciplinary team meetings), and how much inpatient work would be involved to complete this amount of work. The team would also understand what other functions must be completed by the team that are not explicit within the contract. Perhaps the training and teaching commitment to trainees and other specialist services, audit and quality improvement initiatives, research projects, service developments, clinical governance, mandatory training, continuing professional development of each individual, and perhaps *even* team development. The team needs to decide which functions must be the responsibility of the whole team and which functions can be given to individuals or sub-teams.

3) The team would be able to translate this into roles and responsibilities—who does what, and how is this decided? Role allocation would hopefully be shared equitably and in a manner that plays to the strengths of the team. How and when team decisions might be made would be clear and transparent. Who is leading the team and how will they be led? How will conflict be managed? What will be the ground rules for the team and how will they be decided? What will it be like to work in this team? What will be the team culture and mentality? Within this culture, what will the interpersonal relationships be like? How often will the team meet? How will they meet? Will the meeting be 'agenda driven' or 'outcome driven'?

4) Who will the team interact with?

a) Patients

Obviously, central to all that we do are our patients. How will this team interact with patients? How can we best serve their needs? How can we provide the best service? What would success look like? How do we ensure quality? How do we keep up with demand to achieve a timely service?

What would our patients and their relatives say about our team of colorectal surgeons? What would they say about the micro-culture they have generated?

In no particular order for the other interactions are:

b) Clinic teams

c) Theatre teams

d) Wards

e) MDTs

f) Other specialties and professional groups

g) Secretaries

h) Operational manager(s)

i) Clinical director/group director/medical director

j) Other

With each of categories (b) to (j), how would the team interact with each of these other groups/teams/sub-teams? What would success look like in this interaction? How will we know this team is doing a good job? What would the other groups say about our team of colorectal surgeons?

Example 4.3 starts to illustrate that success is not measured by how well the team can run a team meeting but by how well it runs an effective, caring, high-quality, timely service for the patients which also generates positive interactions with all of the other staff groups with which it interacts along the way.

Easy, eh?

Now that I have removed my tongue from where it was lodged firmly in my cheek, we will look more practically at things that might go wrong. Not surprisingly, juggling everything is not at all straightforward so I want offer some thoughts about why teams might not be functioning well together.

Dysfunctions of a team

The classic model that is used to discuss this is Patrick Lencione's five signs of team dysfunction:[11]

1. Absence of trust

2. Fear of conflict

3. Lack of commitment

4. Avoidance of accountability

5. Inattention to results

1. Lencione suggests that the first problem stems from an unwillingness to show vulnerability within the group. We will return to this as a topic when we look at leadership.

2. The second issue is an ostrich approach of creating artificial harmony in the group or an atmosphere where no-one wants to rock the boat. The elephant in the room goes right on sitting there. *(How many metaphors can you fit into two lines, Debbie?)*

3. The third component happens when there is only superficial agreement amongst the team, leaving them with ambiguity. No-one really takes things forward or takes the bull by the horns.

4. The fourth behaviour results in a lowering of standards. Again this is something we will cover when we talk about leadership. The responsibility needs to be shared across the team. *Cliché alert: only the team can fail!*

When successful, this also translates to watching out for each other's back. If someone else has a heavy workload on a particular day and I've finished what I'm doing, I go and help him/her out. I don't just go and sit in the coffee room or leave early. I can be confident in the belief that all my team will do the same for me as I would do for them as we have already got a trusting relationship. The converse, 'it's not my job', is the negative behaviour that will undermine the team and its standards.

5. The fifth behaviour means that focus is on personal outcomes and self rather than on the team, the task, and the results.

Lencione[11] illustrates this model as a triangle with layer 1, at the bottom, the base layer and the foundation on which to build, being absence of trust and building each of the numbers as a subsequent layer (Figure 4.4).

Hawkins[10] identifies eight activities or behaviours that he calls 'interrupters' for a team that overlaps with Lencione's model but adds a few more dimensions.

This is my understanding of Hawkins' eight interrupters:[10]

1. Not having a shared understanding of the purpose of the team.

2. The 'stuckness' of 'either/or' debates that recur without being resolved. It is worth asking if the right question is being considered.

3. Accountability occurs in silos and isn't shared across the team.

4. Pay back. 'We are going to behave like this because they did it to us first!'

5. Inability to convert agreement into action.

This point emphasizes the difference between a superficial 'yes' versus 'who is going to do what by when' *and* the team is happy with what it has agreed

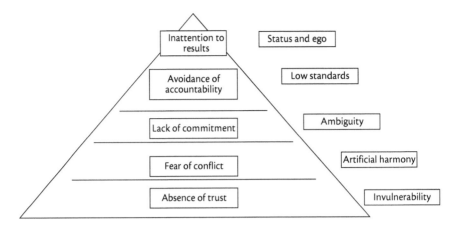

Figure 4.4 The five signs of team dysfunction.
Reproduced with permission from Lencioni P, 2002, *The five dysfunctions of a team*. Oxford: John Wiley and Sons. Copyright © 2002 John Wiley and Sons.

to and people are sufficiently engaged in the process to see it through; i.e. they are committed.

6. The loss of value addition with 'agenda-driven' rather than 'outcome-driven' meetings.

7. The absence of understanding that the success of the team is dependent on the functioning of the team with all of those groups that we illustrated in Example 4.3, not on a 'happy team meeting'.

8. Hawkins uses the metaphor 'ignoring the smell of the dead fish'. I tend to use either the group behaviour of 'ignoring the smell of smoke' or 'failing to name the elephant in the room'. All three metaphors work to acknowledge the fact that there is somehow an unspoken rule in the team not to mention 'subject x'.

What is your team like?

Chances are that you may work in more than one team or the team may have different people on different days. If you consider the most stable team that you work in, how are you doing with each of those five layers of the Lencione triangle? What if we look at all of the eight behaviours that Hawkins describes—is it drafty when you consider any of those?

What developmental needs might your team have? How might you tackle them? Who might you need to help you? How will you go about that? When will you start? What barriers might be in the way? How could you get around those?

With those things in mind, now consider asking yourself and when you are brave enough, consider asking your team:

What might your team need to keep doing but also develop and improve?

What might your team need to stop doing?

What might your team need to start doing?

Back to conflict

I mentioned at the beginning of the chapter that conflict could have a positive effect in promoting change and moving things forward, so I wanted to finish on this more positive aspect. Lencione suggests that *fear* of conflict results in a dysfunctional team, so how do we 'do' conflict safely?

Positive conflict

Eisenhardt[12] found that some successful teams actually seem to thrive on conflict. She explored the common themes within successful teams about the way that they make conflict 'safe' and productive. These were her findings of things to maintain within the team when using positive conflict:

- Common goals
- Focus on the issues not the people
- Fairness
- Option generation to enrich debate
- Keep the power balanced within the group
- Use humour
- Do not force consensus

Key points (up to and including Chapter 4)

- Situational awareness can be considered via three components:
  - Perception (*what?*),
  - comprehension (*so what?*), and
  - predicting future state (*what next?*).
- We make sense of what we have perceived so that it becomes a working mental model.

◆ When working in a team it is important that the ***mental model*** is shared with, and shared by, the team members.

◆ Remember that ***commentating*** is a skill where we voice our thoughts out loud. This not only slows our thinking down and makes it more deliberate, it helps to control our stress levels and it helps others to understand what we thinking. The latter links to generating a shared mental model.

◆ This shared mental model builds towards a team situational assessment or problem definition.

◆ Barriers to perception and comprehension include:

  ◆ high workload,

  ◆ time pressure,

  ◆ perceived high risk,

  ◆ stress,

  ◆ fatigue,

  ◆ biases (including expectation, confirmation, and environmental), and

  ◆ task fixation.

◆ When building our mental model problems can arise due to:

  ◆ missed cues,

  ◆ misinterpreting cues, or

  ◆ choosing to ignore cues,

  ◆ incorrect risk assessment,

  ◆ poor time judgement, or

  ◆ a failure to update our mental model either when new information becomes available or when conditions change.

◆ It can be useful to run through ***SHEEP*** to help with situational awareness.

  ◆ S—Which guideline/SOP are we using? Do we have all of the information we need?

  ◆ H—Who is doing what? How is that working? Is someone time keeping?

- ◆ E—Are we in the best place for what we are dealing with?

- ◆ E—Do we have all the kit that we need?

- ◆ P—How full is my bucket? Where is my focus?

◆ Once we have completed our situational assessment or problem definition we move on to *'what are we going to do about it?'*

◆ There are four main types of decision-making process:

- ◆ *recognition-primed or intuitive,*

- ◆ *rule-based,*

- ◆ *option generation*, and

- ◆ *creative*

◆ How we decide which method suits the situation depends on time pressure, risk, and the novelty of the situation.

◆ The rule-based approach for emergencies exists to make life easier for us.

◆ When we have more time we can use an option-generation model such as DECIDE.

◆ Making a decision is only the first step in a cycle. We should then continuously monitor that treatment or plan and review it. This is especially true in the light of new information.

◆ It is vital to update our mental model with new information.

◆ Please guard against the *assumption* that a given diagnosis is both correct and fixed (correct across all time).

◆ We need to spend more time reviewing how we are making our decisions so that we can improve this skill.

◆ Conflict can be considered as an unmet need.

◆ Conflict can be classed as substantive or personal.

◆ Substantive conflict has a place in change or in moving things forward; it isn't always negative.

◆ It is worth understanding the conflict triangle: people—who is fighting and where are the clashes; process—how does the conflict/the underlying problem manifest itself; problem—what are they fighting about?

- When personal conflict occurs, in understanding the people aspect, it is worth unpicking why conflict has occurred and trying to understand it in terms of MBTI styles, preferred learning styles (Honey and Mumford), and preferred team roles (Belbin).

- When helping to resolve conflict some basic tools are useful; listening skills, open questioning, an understanding of eye contact, posture, stillness, and planning the environment.

- The next important skill is mastering your 'attention'. Improvement with this skill can be helped with mindfulness.

- Other skills that are useful to develop in these settings are self-awareness, self-management, and the management of your own value and belief systems.

- Other skills to acquire include summarizing, reflecting back, positive reframing, hypothesis, pre-framing, prompts, clarifying questions, and appreciative enquiry.

- A mediator may be necessary and very helpful in resolving some conflicts.

- Some of the additional tools a mediator may use include 'normalizing', 'mutualizing', past-to-future state, concatenation, and a skilful use of positive reframing methods.

- Hierarchy management has an important role in conflict resolution.

- The graded assertiveness tool: CUSS (concern, unsure, safety, and stop) can be useful when you need to highlight a concern but don't know quite how to tackle the subject.

- Once conflict has been resolved, there needs to be some time invested in developing the team.

- Coaching has a role to play in both individual and team development.

- A commonly used approach in coaching is TGROW (topic, goal, reality, options, and wrap up/will).

- When considering team development it can be helpful to use Hawkins' approach: CLEAR (contracting, listening, exploring, action, and review).

- Hawkins suggests that the team looks at external fit, internal focus, how they will work together, and who else will the team work with.

- ◆ Lencione suggest there are five main causes of a dysfunctional team:
  - ◆ Absence of trust
  - ◆ Fear of conflict
  - ◆ Lack of commitment
  - ◆ Avoidance of accountability
  - ◆ Inattention to results

References

1. Belbin M. *Management Teams*. London: Heinemann, 2001.
2. Honey P and Mumford A. *The Learning Styles Questionnaire: 80-item version*. Maidenhead: Peter Honey Publications, 2006.
3. Beer J and Packard C. *The Mediator's Handbook*. Gabriola Island, BC, Canada: New Society Publishers, 2012.
4. Whitmore J. *Coaching for Performance* 4th edition. London: Nicholas Brealey. 2009.
5. Walters A. *Crew Resource Management is No Accident*. Wallingford: Aries, 2002.
6. Miller G. The Magical Number Seven, Plus or Minus Two: Some Limits on our Capacity for Processing Information. *Psychological Review* 1956; 63: 81–97.
7. Heifetz R. *Leadership Without Easy Answers*. Cambridge, MA: Belknap Press of Harvard University Press, 1994.
8. Whatling T. *Mediation Skills and Strategies*. Philadelphia, PA: Jessica Kingsley Publishers, 2012.
9. Goleman D. What Makes a Leader? *Harvard Business Review* 1998; 76(6): 93–102.
10. Hawkins P. *Coaching, Mentoring and Organizational Consultancy*. Milton Keynes: Open University Press, 2006.
11. Lencione P. *The Five Dysfunctions of a Team*. Chichester: John Wiley and Sons, 2002.
12. Eisenhardt KM, Kahwajy JL, Bourgeois LJ, 3rd. How Management Teams can have a Good Fight. *Harvard Business Review* 1997; 75(4): 77–85.

5

Debriefing

For the mind does not require filling like a bottle, but rather, like wood, it only requires kindling to create in it an impulse to think independently and an ardent desire for the truth.

Plutarch, AD 46–120

Introduction

Debriefing is a term that is used to refer to a number of different forms of what I'm going to refer to as a 'learning conversation'. You can also think of it as 'post-event analysis'. I find that using the term 'debriefing' on the shop floor can alienate people, so when you introduce it to your team I suggest you find your own term for the process that the team feels it can own (examples include 'wash up', 'huddle', 'chat', or it can be done as part of handover).

Historically, the term seems to have originated in the military where it referred to a group of people talking through their experience in battle after an event in order to capture any other information that may be useful. This information was then used to plan subsequent interactions.

The term has also been adopted by psychologists. Here it refers to the activity of exploring the emotions generated by and the impact of a traumatic event. Debriefing in this setting, as a therapeutic intervention, is most definitely the realm of a trained clinical psychologist and is not something to be dabbled in by well-meaning health professionals.

Debriefing forms a regular part of the processes incorporated in aviation.

In educational settings, debriefing at the end of an event can be used to capture learning. This may occur following an actual or a simulated 'acute' episode. (Acute in this sense, and throughout the book, will be used to refer to a sudden or short-term event. The opposite is chronic, which refers to something long term.)

However, debriefing doesn't have to be something that is associated with an acute event or when something has gone wrong. There is also the daily debrief which will hopefully become routine across healthcare, where at the end of a shift or day a short conversation takes place which highlights areas of good practice. It is also a forum for delivering praise and searching for any improvements that can be made to current practice. It is a conversational style approach to making little tweaks to what we do so that we generate continuous improvement and ensure that we are not complacent.

Debriefing can be performed for one individual (e.g. if someone was unsuccessful at interview), or take place in a group (e.g. following a cardiac arrest or on completion of a project).

Whilst there are underlying principles that underpin all of these activities, there are also some fairly big differences.

The next section will highlight the debriefing practices that are most relevant to everyday use in healthcare. I will then introduce a series of simple rules and tips that can be used across the board for different purposes. I will highlight some of the aspects to consider when facilitating a group debriefing session rather than working with an individual.

Debriefing in formal settings, such as after a traumatic event, needs specialist skills. As I mentioned earlier, there is a specific tool—a psychological debrief— that is suitable for use only by clinical psychologists or similar professionals. I will not be discussing this here. I want to emphasize that there is a spectrum of debriefing required for different settings and to encourage us all to consider where our limits might be and when we might need expert help, such as a clinical psychologist or simply someone with more experience than ourselves.

To become skilled at facilitating a 'group debrief' takes a lot of practice. A daily mini debriefing or wash up, however, should be able to be run by anyone leading a team.

Educational theory

If it is learning that we are looking for, then it makes sense to spend a bit of time reviewing how adults learn. I am going to offer a nutshell version here as a quick summary.

I want to revisit Honey and Mumford[1] and their 80-point questionnaire. This is something that I recommend you complete. The results can be plotted on two intersecting axes. The north–south axis represents the learning spectrum of activist to theorist. The east–west axis represents the spectrum of pragmatist to reflector.

When you plot your results you will end up with some sort of quadrilateral. In an ideal world you would be able to teach and learn via all of the four styles represented (activist, theorist, pragmatist, and reflector). In reality, you will usually have two preferred styles of learning and two that you might need to spend a bit of time developing! There is no right or wrong style. The idea is that to learn fully, you need to master all four styles.

When you teach you will find it easiest to teach in your preferred learning style. In order to master teaching a mixed group with different learners, you will need to learn to teach in all four styles too. We will explore this in more detail later.

Honey and Mumford: Using a camera metaphor

The way I usually ask people to work out which style they lean towards is by using the metaphor of a camera.

I want you to imagine that I have just been incredibly generous and given you a camera! I want you to think about what you would do with it.

There are a group of learners who would just take it out of the box and start pressing the buttons to see what happened. This group might be considered to fall into the Honey and Mumford group, activists.

A different group might like to find out from someone else what the different buttons do and how these might be useful (i.e. the practical applications). After finding these things out, they would happily experiment on their own. These would fall broadly into the group called pragmatists.

Another group would take out the manual and read that first before touching the camera. These would be theorists.

The final group might not touch the camera at all yet and just consider first the concept of photography. These would be reflectors.

As part of your self-awareness, do you know your preferred learning style? If not, can you hazard a guess? Which types of learning would you find least rewarding and which most challenging?

Any debrief of a group of individuals will probably involve participants with these different styles. As a debrief is all about generating a *learning conversation*, you will ideally need to be aware of how each individual likes to learn, and you will need to cover all of those styles.

Double-loop learning

I want to introduce the concept described by Chris Argyris[2-7] to challenge the way we think about experiences and how we learn from them. The reason that I am referring to this in the debriefing section is because it is precisely this double-loop learning that we can achieve with an effective debrief.

The single loop

Step 1

If we imagine a step-wise progression around a circle, the first step represents us 'doing something'. We can refer to this 'doing something' as an activity or process or action. It could be our current practice or simply how we did that activity today.

Step 2

The next step might be identifying any errors that we made or reviewing any mistakes.

Step 3

We now change the action. This involves providing solutions and planning the changes.

And repeat

Start again at step 1.

This is single-loop learning. We simply try to do the same thing better.

The double-loop

Step 4

Within step 3 we introduce an extra step. This takes a deeper look at the error and tries to explore why it happened. Argyris encourages us to explore 'governing values'. These values underpin the ways that we think and behave. He encourages us to question assumptions, consider other perspectives, and unpick our defensive responses that may be causing us to continue doing something the same way. He challenges us to look at why we tend to stick with processes that are not effective and why we have not challenged ourselves on this. This second loop can be considered in a similar way to taking the balcony view that we have discussed earlier.

A skilled debrief is a brilliant way to have these challenging conversations.

A bit of history in medical education

When I first started working in education we were told that we had to say seven positive things to someone before we could say something negative. I was taught to put my hand in my pocket and count them on my fingers as I trotted out all my positive comments. As you know, I am still a great fan of praise and positive feedback but now I'd rather it wasn't delivered in an artificial dollop. I would like it to be real not forced.

When I attended my first instructor's course I was introduced to Pendleton's feedback model,[8] This model, which was used extensively in resuscitation courses, went something along the lines of:

1. tell me what went well.

2. now I will tell you what I thought went well.

3. tell me what you could have done better.

4. now I will tell you how I think you should improve.

The result of the combination of these was that if someone wanted to start by being negative about his or her own performance, it just wasn't allowed. We were taught to stop them from being negative and instead get them to start with the positives. This principle was applied even if it was a teaching scenario and the whole thing had been a bit of a 'train wreck'.

If I am brutally honest there were days when the resuscitation teaching case staff had just attempted had gone so badly that it was really hard to think of lots of positive things to say. I would struggle at that time to maintain my belief in the person I was training (I like to think I'm better at this now with 20 years of practice).

I think it is also quite characteristically British to focus on the negatives and want to be perfect. It is very common for people's first thoughts to be about what didn't work well, or about something they forgot to do, or the fact that it took them a long time to achieve a particular task.

Time has moved on. We are going to let people say what they want to say and not be so parental about it.

There may be another feedback model with which you are familiar.

The sandwich feedback model

This is sometimes known as the positive–negative–positive sandwich or it can be called a … (*rude word*) sandwich. (The rude word might medically be described as faeces but it is the more colloquial expletive equivalent!)

The idea stemmed from the fact that people were quite scared of giving negative feedback so they would hide the unpalatable bit by covering it up with praise on either side.

We are going to move on to explore some of the more modern thoughts on debriefing. The idea is to develop a learning conversation. This moves away from judgement. It moves away from positive and negative. It moves away from what went well or what could be improved. It moves away from right and wrong. It moves away from polarization.

The focus is on learning.

We can learn from things that have gone well in just the same way as we can learn from an error, but this has been a less common experience in most of the educational environments I know.

Traditionally, if there is a problem, there may well be a conversation (often a blame-based conversation) about *who* has done *what* wrong and about how they shouldn't do it again.

How often do you unpick something that has gone really well? What were the key things that made a real difference today?

Open questions and appreciative enquiry

We are going to re-introduce these two techniques that we have already covered in the conflict, mediation, and coaching sections.

There should be mostly open questions, with a few clarifying questions here and there.

I would suggest that the person doing the debrief should only be talking 20 per cent of the time. We call this the 80:20 rule. In a more inexperienced group it may be necessary to slip into a teaching mode briefly, before moving back into debriefing mode. In a really experienced group, people may almost debrief themselves and the facilitator can be even more hands off.

It is a good question to ask yourself as you go along, what are the talking ratios here?

The process of the debrief, for me, should be like the coaching model; almost invisible to those you are debriefing. It should be possible to steer the debrief in a particular direction by asking good questions. Again, I like to stimulate thought and reflection.

I am going to stick with the educational debrief—either post simulation or at the end of day for some learning or after a routine event. (For now, I want to avoid the debrief in which we suspect there is psychological distress.)

The coat hanger for the debrief: A traffic cone

Apologies for the mixed metaphor. Let's hope I can unpick it! I think it is always good to have something on which to hang your debrief (I tend to think of it as a coat hanger). There are many models available[9] and mine is an adaptation of a common one.

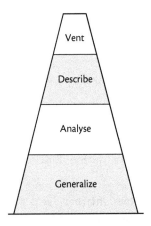

Figure 5.1 The traffic-cone model.

There are four phases. They remind me of a traffic cone. It starts narrow and gets broader as it goes down. My first traffic cone has four stripes. Subsequent traffic cones have three stripes. And then there is a closure phase.

I tend to think of a debrief as a line of traffic cones (see Figures 5.1 and 5.2).

The first four phases are:

1. Vent

2. Description

3. Analysis

4. Generalization/Application

This can be represented with the acronym VDAG.

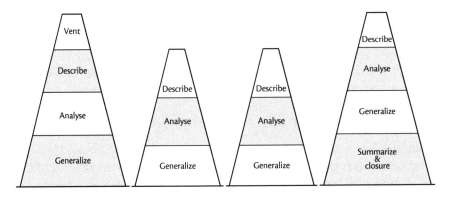

Figure 5.2 The row of traffic cones.

The vent phase allows people to get things off their chest. This moves to a description of part of what happened. The person who is being debriefed will choose what to focus on here, not the facilitator. The facilitator will help to make sense of what has happened in the analysis phase and start to bring in other members of the group in a safe way. This will move on to introducing parallel experiences, and finally looking how this learning can be used to influence future practice.

So the overall pattern might be VDAG, DAG, DAG, closure (see Figure 5.2). There may be more occurrences of the DAG depending on how much time there is and how many points you wish to raise in the debrief.

What I am not advocating is that you describe the whole thing, then analyse the whole thing, and then generalize the whole thing. I will return to why as we go along.

V: Venting

I usually start off with an open question like 'so, how was that?' And then I listen. Active listening, as covered in Chapter 4. Listening and watching not only for what is said, but how it is said, and what is not said, looking for the non-verbal cues as well as hearing the verbal ones, and not only from the person you are asking but non-verbal cues from the rest of the group as well.

The next steps and what you are going to say will be reactive. You cannot plan them in advance, which is why it is harder to learn. It depends what has been said. There needs to be acknowledgment and perhaps some of the summarizing or reflecting back skills employed that we covered in Chapter 3.

I would also recommend the SAGE & THYME® model for dealing with distress. This is a level 1 communication skills course that is suitable for everyone in healthcare and gives you a safe way to manage distress should it occur. The model uses each of the letters as a mnemonic. The first half of the model encourages you to think about where you might talk, enquire whether someone would like to talk, and gather all of the issues whilst displaying empathy. The second half of the model asks people who they usually talk to when they are distressed and how these help before encouraging people to consider what other help they need. The aim, like a coaching approach, is to leave the responsibility for solving the problem with its owner.

There can be emotion involved when people feel that they have made an error or missed something in front of their peer group. Use of the SAGE & THYME® model is a helpful skill to have up your sleeve to feel equipped to handle this.

If we are ready to move on to the next phase, then we need a way to link to it seamlessly: a link sentence.

D—Description

If there has been only one topic offered up in the vent then this might be explored in a bit more depth. A link sentence might be something like 'tell me more about that.'

If there were multiple topics covered in the vent then it is worth asking which of those people would like to cover first, or choosing the one you think has the most significance.

The link sentence might be something along the lines of 'so what I think I've heard you say is ... and something about ... Which of those shall we talk about first?'

The individual answers. You might follow this with, 'so, talk me through that bit in more detail.'

Once you feel you have a good description of the particular event, you can start to link towards the analysis phase.

A—Analyse

'So what were your thoughts at that time?', or

'How did you come to that decision?', or

'Unpick that for me', or

'What was going on for you then?', or

'What was that like?'

Once the analysis is starting to flow, I like to broaden it to the group or the other faculty members if you have a fellow debriefer.

'Other thoughts?', with an opening-of-hands gesture to encourage others to participate.

If the group hasn't warmed up yet, consider using hypotheses (see Chapter 4) to get the ball rolling.

'When I was watching ... I found myself wondering ... What are your thoughts on that?'

This highlights the double-loop learning or the balcony view that we mentioned earlier.

Once the analysis has enough substance, it is time to go the wider part of the traffic cone and to broaden the topic.

G—Generalize

This phase can also be known as the application phase: how will you apply the learning in the future?

To the group or other facilitator you might say, 'can someone share a parallel experience?' or 'what have people come across that might be similar?' If nothing is volunteered and I think it would benefit the person to know they are not alone with what they have just done, I will share one of my own stories. I think it helps to demonstrate some vulnerability from the debriefer and it adds to the psychological safety of the session. We will all make mistakes, it is important to act as a good role model and demonstrate an open culture. It also helps to level off the hierarchy and helps people to feel we are not there to sit in judgement on them.

I also 'normalize' (see 'normalizing' in Chapter 4) at this phase, if I think it would be useful. I think there is a place for making sure that the environment is a safe one to make mistakes.

I often introduce a cognitive aid at this point if I have had time ('here's one I prepared earlier!' And yes, I think the careful use of humour in a debrief is useful to create an informal and relaxed learning environment. Obviously there are times when this approach is not appropriate). This could be the relevant guideline for the scenario or the G-NO-TECS tool if an issue about non-technical skills is being raised.

By now the emphasis is very much on a general conversation about principles. It is no longer about what one person did or didn't do, nor the specifics of what has happened that day.

We then need to make the link to future state. 'How might we use this?' Once the application of the learning has been established and explored, I then repeat the DAG process.

In a simulation session debrief, I try to select any important technical issues that have arisen plus highlight two aspects of the non-technical skills for each scenario. As far as the length of the debrief goes, it is thought best to aim for a ratio of one part scenario to two parts debrief. If you are doing a daily debrief I realize you won't have the luxury of this amount of time.

Once the last traffic cone reaches the stage of establishing the future state, I encourage a final stage of reflection. I ask each member of the group to share something that he or she will take away from the session. This serves more than one purpose. Not only does it help to encourage a bit more thinking and cementing but it gives me feedback about what the learning has been about. It is possible to consider the balance between the technical and non-technical learning and to do what I call a 'rocking-horse dropping check'. If there has been a massive gap in knowledge/skills/non-technical skills identified but it isn't mentioned in this closure phase, it gives you another bite at the cherry. It is possible to redirect the session and go over what you think is important and perhaps tackle it from another direction. You can then check understanding before you move on or finish the session.

The tools

What we have covered so far is simply the framework for the process. Now we need to consider the tools we might employ within a debrief session.

The following tools are vital to a debrief, and have already been discussed in Chapter 4: active listening, open questions (avoid the double question), appreciative enquiry, praise (consider delivering it using SBIC to make it more meaningful), and the use of silence. I also like to use humour when it's appropriate to break the ice and lift the mood. This may involve laughing at myself. I think fun is an essential part of a learning environment.

The next tools are really useful but not essential and were also covered in Chapter 4: hypothesis, summarizing, reflecting back, positive reframing, 'normalizing', paraphrasing, use of metaphor, and pre-framing.

The 80:20 rule encourages us to remember that the person we are debriefing should be doing most of the talking. I tend to think of the facilitator as just nudging the conversation along. An experienced group will almost debrief themselves but they might need to be encouraged to name a few elephants in the room. A less experienced group might need some sections where the facilitator switches to instructing briefly before switching back to facilitation.

You cannot pre-plan the questions you are going to ask. Novice facilitators find this difficult to grasp. You need to follow the thread of the participants which involves lots of listening. Only once you have listened and processed can you form your question. This takes practice. You can introduce topics that you think are important (perhaps one or two technical and one or two non-technical issues). It is important that the questioning techniques don't stay at a superficial level. The technique that I call 'layering' encourages you to dig a bit deeper. This involves engaging in your best active listening mode, processing what has been said, and then selecting a question that probes what has been said in more detail. There are some simple phrases that can help.

'Tell me more about that?'

'How did that come about?'

'What was happening for you at that time?'

'What led you to that conclusion?'

'How did you make that decision?'

Look out for the body language that tells you that you have asked a good question that has provoked thought. It usually is met with a pause (for thinking time). The person may adopt a 'thinking face'—we are all different but you usually lose eye contact for a bit. There is a balancing act at this point. You need to wait and use silence and know the difference between thinking, floundering, and being completely lost, switching to 'bunny in the headlights' as they can't think of an answer. Remember to keep it safe, if people struggle to find an answer be prepared to 'fill' with a hypothesis or a rewording of the question. If you do the latter take responsibility for having not asked the question very well.

We need to plan the environment for the debrief. I usually recommend a circle layout with facilitators mixed in with the group to create a fraternal feel—'we are all learning together'. This makes it easier to get the conversation flowing around the group. It is sometimes a challenge to get everyone involved in the debrief but it is a worthy aim. It is important to establish whether someone who is quiet is very reflective or whether there is hierarchy or past experiences with others in the room. The person may simply not be engaged, or perhaps they fear saying something stupid or being judged. I do not use the 'name and shame' method to force them to say something. I also try to avoid 'death by circle' where everyone *must have a turn.* I do try to encourage them with body language: gentle eye contact or an inviting hand gesture. I find silence helpful. I may also tease people about how interesting the floor looks when they are trying to avoid my gaze, but this would always be directed at the group and not at a specific individual.

We need to create a feeling of psychological safety. This is partly achieved with a pre-brief in a simulation session, but the issue needs to be handled in the introduction to the debrief if it is happening after an actual event. It is important to create an open atmosphere where people feel able to talk about mistakes. They need to feel they are not being judged either by the facilitators or by their peer group. They need to feel they are not the only person who has ever made a mistake; we all make them. The emphasis should be on the learning. Others (including facilitators) should be encouraged to share mistakes and learning. Story-telling in this setting can be a useful tool.

Avoid some of the clichéd phrases like:

> How would you do it differently next time?
>
> What could you improve on …?

Both of these phrases have a negative and judgemental tone.

Try replacing them with something about learning, like:

> What will you take away with you today?
>
> What have you learnt?

What is the most important thing you learned today?

How will you be able to use this in the future?

What questions have you been left with?

If it is a simulation that has gone wrong and the person seems intent on self-flagellation, it can be worth giving them another bite at the cherry. You can offer them the chance to replay the simulation and let them reinforce the new learning by putting it into practice. This also has the added benefit of lifting their spirits before they leave.

Within the debrief the facilitators must maintain self-awareness and self-management (focused attention, emotional intelligence), and maintain belief in the people they are debriefing. By this, I mean 'believe' that they are competent and usually good at their job but that perhaps nerves got the better of them today or that the stress of being watched overfilled their bucket.

It is important for the facilitator to spend some time on the balcony looking at his or her self-management.

Body language is something that we have touched on, but remember eye contact, posture, head nodding (but not like a 'Churchillian' dog), and the layout of the room helps to influence how close you are, physically and emotionally. Think about your 'interested' face and how you might exhibit empathy, but also how you might take control of a situation to change direction if appropriate. There are a few professional groups where I have found it necessary to rein in the feedback from peers when it gets too brutal. Have a plan for how you might achieve this.

It can also be important to stop one or two people from dominating the session. 'Someone else with some thoughts?' 'Has anyone else got something they would like to add?' 'Anyone got a different perspective?' 'Anyone come across something like this before?' Accompany this with trying to make eye contact around the room and an open hand gesture.

There are some other behavioural challenges that you might face in debriefing. In a simulation session one of those is colloquially known as 'simulatoritis'. This is where participants struggle to buy into the reality of the scenario, but this can also be an excuse for not wishing to own up to errors and blaming mistakes and problems on the manikin. It is important to acknowledge shortcomings of manikins in the pre-briefing and, for example, to acknowledge that their breathing sounds aren't perfect. But it is also important to relate some of these things to real life: 'does anyone think we ever struggle to pick up on physical signs in real life?' This can stimulate a discussion and highlight some learning points.

There is another behaviour that is also peculiar to being in simulation: hyper-vigilance. The participant checks things over and over again, just waiting for the 'thing to go wrong'. I see it regularly with anaesthetic trainees who try everything to delay actually giving the anaesthetic in the scenario as they assume that is when something terrible will happen. They can sometimes get themselves so worried that what is a perfectly simple grade 1 intubation (and I have changed nothing at all on the manikin) becomes a failed intubation and difficult airway simply because that is what they are expecting to happen. I think this offers a great opportunity in the debrief to talk about the boxing gloves of stress, how full your bucket is, and the two-breath technique. It needs to be handled sensitively so that people don't feel undermined. I make sure I 'normalize' strongly. I take responsibility for the stressful environment. I suggest that simulation often raises our adrenalin levels. I then move the focus to learning about how to recognize stress and how to deal with it. I make sure I generalize for the whole group to take pressure off the person in the hot seat.

I can't emphasize enough the importance of learning through laughter and fun. I think these are useful countermeasures, or coping strategies, for stress (with the caveats already mentioned).

After-action review

I want to introduce you to one more framework for use after an event, the after-action review. This could, however, also be used to frame your simple daily debrief.[10]

It consists of four questions:[10]

1. What was expected to happen?

2. What actually happened?

3. Why is there a difference between these?

4. What has been learned?

I like this simply framework from Cronin and Andrews.[10] I might modify the third question slightly to remove the word 'why', as it can appear too aggressive a question and may inhibit a reply. I would also personalize some of the questions.

My version would be subtly different and I would add a further question:

1. **What did you expect to happen?**

2. **What actually happened?**

3. **What are the differences between these?**

4. **How do you think they came about? Consider SHEEP.**

5. **What have we learned?**

By using this framework the focus becomes looking at whether people had the same expectations from the beginning. It is important that everyone has a say.

When they get to the equivalent of the descriptive phase, it will be important to think about the different perspectives that there are held by the people in the room and the defensive responses that might be influencing how people are making sense of a situation in retrospect. Some of the skills that we discussed in conflict resolution ('normalizing' and 'mutualizing') may be relevant in this setting.

Creating a feeling of psychological safety will be paramount. I think it is also important to be able to spot cues indicating people who might benefit from psychological support. We oughtn't to try to tackle this ourselves in an amateur way; just because we are in healthcare doesn't mean we are all skilled psychologists. It is important to understand our boundaries and capabilities and to know when to refer on for other more specialist help.

The framework gives you sections to use. I might introduce it at the beginning of the session when I'm trying to go through how the session might work. The conversation might run as follows: 'So, as we discussed, I'm keen to get to grips with what everyone thought should be happening, your expectations. Can we hear from each of you about what you expected to happen that day?' If no-one starts to talk, I might add: 'Would someone like to start us off?' Then I might use some silence. There is no completely formulaic approach. A facilitator should do what feels natural and the session should be tailor-made for the group. The words I've used here are simply examples, not a prescriptive plan. The framework gives you the overall headings to work with.

Dealing with an event is different from a daily debrief. If you were doing a routine daily 'wash up' you could simply ask the questions as they are, without settling everyone in and spending time establishing a safe environment. It could just be a much more informal chat at the end of a session or shift.

The purpose of the debrief is learning

The debrief that we have been discussing here is not the psychology model; it is the model for promoting double-loop learning. It is a fantastic tool for raising awareness, for questioning assumptions, for challenging perspectives and causing a healthy challenge to the status quo. It can be used to aid the acquisition of knowledge and skills and to explore attitudes and behaviours.

I am going to finish this chapter on a soap box (Box 5.1).

Box 5.1 Soap-box moment

I believe we should be doing a miniature debriefing every day and a longer version as often as we can. I think everyone in a leadership role should have the skills to run a debrief effectively. If we were to address this, a number of our current leaders would need to work hard on increasing their emotional intelligence (EQ).

Key points (up to and including Chapter 5)

◆ Situational awareness can be broken down into three components:

  ◆ Perception (*what?*),

  ◆ comprehension (*so what?*), and

  ◆ predicting future state (*what next?*).

◆ We make sense of what we have perceived so that it becomes a working mental model.

◆ When working in a team it is important that the ***mental model*** is shared with, and shared by, the team members.

◆ Remember that ***commentating*** is a skill where we talk our thoughts aloud. This not only slows our thinking down and makes it more deliberate, it helps to control our stress levels and it helps others to understand what we are thinking. The latter links to generating a shared mental model.

◆ This shared mental model builds towards a team situational assessment or problem definition.

◆ Barriers to perception and comprehension include:

  ◆ high workload,

  ◆ time pressure,

  ◆ perceived high risk,

  ◆ stress,

  ◆ fatigue,

  ◆ biases (including expectation, confirmation, and environmental), and

  ◆ task fixation.

◆ When building our mental model problems can arise due to:

  ◆ missed cues,

  ◆ misinterpreting cues, or

  ◆ choosing to ignore cues,

  ◆ incorrect risk assessment,

  ◆ poor time judgement, or

- a failure to update our mental model either when new information becomes available or when conditions change.
- It can be useful to run through **SHEEP** to help with situational awareness.
  - S—which guideline/SOP are we using? Do we have all of the information we need?
  - H—who is doing what? How is that working? Is someone time keeping?
  - E—are we in the best place for what we are treating?
  - E—do we have all the kit that we need?
  - P—how full is my bucket? Where is my focus?
- Once we have completed our situational assessment or problem definition we move on to '*what are we going to do about it?*'
- There are four main types of decision-making process:
  - *recognition-primed or intuitive,*
  - *rule-based,*
  - *option generation,* and
  - *creative.*
- How we decide which method suits the situation depends on time pressure, risk and the newness of the situation
- The rule-based approach for emergencies exists to make life easier for us.
- When we have more time we can use an option-generation model such as DECIDE.
- Making a decision is only the first step in a cycle. We should then continuously monitor that treatment or plan and review it. This is especially true in the light of new information being presented.
- It is vital to update our mental model with new information.
- Please guard against the *assumption* that the diagnosis is definitely correct.
- We need to spend more time reviewing how we are making our decisions so that we can improve this skill.
- Conflict can be considered as an **unmet need**.
- Conflict can be classed as substantive or personal.

- Substantive conflict has a place in change or in moving things forward. It isn't always negative.

- It is worth understanding the conflict triangle: people—who is fighting and where the clashes are; process—how the conflict manifests itself; and the underlying problem itself—what they are fighting about.

- When personal conflict occurs, in understanding the people aspect, it is worth unpicking why it has occurred and trying to understand it in terms of MBTI styles, preferred learning styles (Honey and Mumford), and preferred team roles (Belbin).

- When helping to resolve conflict some basic tools are useful; listening skills, perfecting your interested and open questioning skills, and an understanding of eye contact, posture, stillness, and planning the environment.

- The next important skill is mastering your 'attention'. Improvement with this skill can be helped with mindfulness.

- Other skills that are useful to develop in these settings are self-awareness, self-management, and the management of your own value and belief system.

- Other skills to acquire include summarizing, reflecting back, positive reframing, hypothesis, pre-framing, prompts, clarifying questions, and appreciative enquiry.

- A mediator may be necessary and very helpful in resolving some conflicts.

- Some of the additional tools a mediator may use include 'normalizing', 'mutualizing', past-to-future state, concatenation, and a skilful use of positive reframing.

- Hierarchy management has an important role in conflict resolution.

- The graded assertiveness tool CUSS can be useful when you need to highlight a concern but don't know quite how to tackle the subject. It stands for Concern, Unsure, Safety, and Stop.

- Once conflict has been resolved, there needs to be some time invested in developing the team.

- Coaching has a role to play in both individual and team development.

- A commonly used approach in coaching is TGROW; Topic, Goal, Reality, Options, and Will/Wrap up.

- When considering team development it can be helpful to use Hawkins' approach CLEAR (Contracting, Listening, Exploring, Action, and Review).

- Hawkins suggests that the team look at external fit, internal focus, how they will work together, and with what other people the team will work.

- Lencione suggests there are five main causes of a dysfunctional team:

  - absence of trust,

  - fear of conflict,

  - lack of commitment,

  - avoidance of accountability, and

  - inattention to results.

- Debriefing helps us achieve double-loop learning.

- Honey and Mumford describe four preferred learning styles: activists, pragmatists, theorists, and reflectors.

- We need to cater for all learning styles.

- There are a number of debriefing models to use as a framework. I use the traffic-cone method of vent, description, analysis, generalize/apply to real situations.

- Useful techniques include 80:20, open questions, appreciative enquiry, use of silence, summarizing, reflect back, hypothesis, pre-framing, para-phrasing, and 'normalizing'.

- We should all aim for a daily debrief, even if we work on our own. 'What did I learn today?' 'How will that change what I do in the future?'

- After-action review is another simple framework.

- My slightly adapted version of the after-action review is:

  - **what did you expect to happen?**

  - **what actually happened?**

  - **what are the differences between these?**

  - **how do you think they came about? Consider SHEEP**

  - **what have we learned?**

References

1. Honey P, Mumford A. *The Learning Styles Questionnaire: 80-item version*. Maidenhead: Peter Honey Publications, 2006.
2. Argyris C. *Understanding Organizational Behaviour*. London: Tavistock Publications, 1960.
3. Argyris C, Schon DA. *Theory in Practice: Increasing Professional Effectiveness*. San Francisco, CA: Jossey-Bass, 1974.
4. Argyris C. *Overcoming Organizational Defenses: Facilitating Organizational learning*. Upper Saddle River; NJ: Pearson Education, 1990.
5. Argyris C, Schon DA. *Organizational Learning II: Theory, Method, and Practice*. Reading, Mass., Wokingham: Addison Wesley, 1996.
6. Argyris C. *On Organizational Learning*, 2nd edn. Oxford: Blackwell Publishers, 1999.
7. Argyris C. *Organizational Traps: Leadership, Culture, Organizational Design*. Oxford: Oxford University Press, 2010.
8. Pendleton D. *The Consultation: An Approach to Learning and Teaching*. Oxford: Oxford University Press, 1984.
9. Fanning RM, Gaba DM. The Role of Debriefing in Simulation-Based Learning. *Simulation in Healthcare* 2007; 2(2): 115–25.
10. Cronin G, Andrews S. After Action Reviews: A New Model for Learning. *Emergency Nurse* 2009; 17(3): 32–5.

6

Leadership

A leader is best when people barely know he exists ... He acts without unnecessary speech, and when the work is done the people say 'We did it ourselves'.

Lao Tzu, *c*.604–*c*.531 BC

Background

Leadership and management comprise a vast field. I want to give you a brief overview of some of the background before bringing things up to date with some of the more recent thinking in the field, and then illustrate the role that human factors has to play in this area. I believe the field of human factors has a lot to offer the field of leadership.

There have been a number of trends in leadership theory over the years (some of them are cyclical). Initially, the trends focused on the individual leader and their characteristics and personality (or 'traits'). This was followed by approaches that looked at behaviours and styles of leadership. The thinking here is that perhaps the key issue was not about a leader's character but instead about how he or she behaved in different situations.

We will start with a rapid canter through trait theory. We will glimpse transactional and transformational leadership. We will consider situational leadership—matching the behaviour or style to the circumstance: you may also have heard it referred to as contingency leadership.

The traditional view of a leader as an all-knowing 'hero' continues to be considered by some as the ideal way they think they should lead. We will consider 'post-heroic' leadership and hopefully convince you that we really should have moved beyond this conception.

Lastly, we will look at more complex social models: adaptive leadership and distributive leadership, and add in some human factors.

Personal characteristics (trait theories): The heroic leaders

As early as the 1920s, people believed that it must be possible to identify common traits in famous leaders. All one had to do to be a great leader oneself was to emulate them (see Exercise 6.1).

Exercise 6.1 Heroic leaders

You will need a pen and paper or a tablet.

I want you to write down the names of five leaders that history would have us believe were great leaders.

How have you chosen your five?

I suspect I would get very different answers if I asked people from different parts of the world, but on a UK-based leadership course there are some regular ones that are usually mentioned. Before I give the names of those away, I want you to look at your list. I want you to look for commonality. Try to make a list of any things that your five people have in common.

Have you listed any leaders who did terrible things but were very effective in getting people to follow their ideas? Or have you gone with people who share admirable goals?

Here is a list of characteristics that are usually offered on a leadership course. I want to make it clear that this is not *my* list. Some traits are controversial and people discuss them to encourage debate (sometimes heated). I want to emphasize again that we are looking at leadership at the moment as the capacity to create a vision, share that vision, and persuade people to follow it. I do not wish to condone what the vision was (I know the word 'vision' can produce eye rolling, so feel free to substitute 'big idea'), nor how the leader went about achieving it. I do not wish to offend anyone but I do want to stimulate you to think. I want you to think broadly; your list could include spiritual as well as business and political leaders.

This list usually includes some of the following people:

Gandhi, Mandela, Mother Teresa, Martin Luther King, Churchill, Thatcher, Hitler, Washington, Florence Nightingale, Lenin, Lincoln, and Shackleton.

What common ground can you find amongst that vastly differing group? Scribble down four similarities before you read on. What do you mean you can't find any similarities between Hitler and Mother Teresa!

(Yes, of course, I am being over reliant on the tongue in my cheek. I wonder sometimes if I am overdoing this form of wit in my general conversations as my daughter, who is five as I write this, seems to be experimenting with it and announcing with great glee that she was being sarcastic! Note to self—perhaps a little more care with my role modelling is required.)

Of course, this is where the trait theories came unstuck: it is very hard to find similarities or common characteristics among such disparate people.

My thoughts on common traits are:

All had a vision or future that they really believed in.

All managed to communicate that vision.

All managed to persuade others to follow that vision.

All could make judgements about a given situation; that is, they could read it.

As far as personal attributes go there may be many more differences than similarities between the leaders you have chosen. A whole range of problems come up, too, when we look at leadership in this way—what role do the followers play in determining leadership traits? What role does circumstance or context play? And what are the 'results' or the impact of their leadership?

Styles and behaviours

If we move on to some other ideas for leadership, we might consider some of the styles of leadership and how leaders might behave in different situations.

In the 1930s, Lewin[1,2] suggested that there are three types of leadership: autocratic, democratic, and laissez-faire. The former was when a leader made a unilateral decision without consulting the team. The democratic style allowed input from the team before making the decision, and the last style involved leaving responsibility for the decision entirely with the team, hence the three styles form a spectrum.

I want you to consider first what it would be like to lead in each of those three styles and then what would it like to be a follower? Which of those styles most closely reflects your own preference?

I want you to imagine you need a group of your peers to agree to a new idea; which of those approaches might be most beneficial? What might be the outcome if you tried to use some of the other styles?

The Blake–Mouton[3] managerial grid uses two axes: concern for people and concern for production. I want to play devil's advocate and substitute the word '*target*' for their equivalent of 'production'.

By classifying types on the axes as either high or low, it is possible to produce a grid with five kinds of managers:

1. Impoverished—low concern for people, low concern for target

2. Country club—high concern for people, low concern for target

3. Produce or perish—high concern for target, low concern for people

4. Team leader—high concern for both

5. Middle of the road—as the name suggests, neither high nor low

Where are you placed and why?

Where is your organization placed and why?

What is it like to work in our target-driven culture?

Where would you like to be?

If you would like to change, what currently prevents you from being where you would like to be? What can you do about that? When could you take the first step? What would that first step be?

A situational approach to styles

As discussed in Level One, Goleman[4] would take this kind of approach. A leader ideally perfects a number of styles and then adjusts the style according to the situation. In the case of Goleman, there is a large emphasis on the sensing that is required to make this work. Only with a well-developed emotional intelligence (EQ) will you be able to sense the situation in the first place and then take the next step of matching the appropriate style for the situation. The five domains of EQ are self-awareness, self-regulation, empathy, motivation, and social skills.

Goleman[4] uses six leadership categories: commanding, visionary, affiliative, democratic, pacesetting, and coaching. These are covered in more depth in Level One (pp. 67–71).

Power as a driver for leadership

French and Raven[5,6] suggest that power and leadership are strongly related and describe five types of power: legitimate (where the person has a hierarchical position), reward (where someone has the ability to offer benefits to another), expert (where there is specialist knowledge or skill), referent (due to the personal attributes of the person), and coercive (where the person is perceived to have the ability to punish).

Which of these causes you to respond well? Are there any that trigger the rebel in you and if so, why is that?

Have you ever been in a meeting where you have seen someone threaten to wield a big stick and it has triggered a mini rebellion not because of the issue at stake itself but because of the leader's behaviour?

Do you know any natural rule-breakers or mavericks? What is it that makes them behave that way? Can you unpick the dynamics of what they are doing and why?

How might you need to modify your delivery so you avoid triggering other people's buttons?

Transactional leadership

In a nutshell, this type of leadership involves the carrot-and-stick approach of reward and punishment. There is an assumption that work is only done because it is rewarded or there is some incentive to do it. It can also be known as managerial leadership. It is thought to be used to maintain the status quo.

Transformational leadership

This approach to leadership is about two key areas—developing a shared vision and inspiring people to work towards it. When the goals and vision are clear and communicated well, the atmosphere in the team is one of encouragement and support. The leader provides a role model for positive behaviour and is inspiring and honest. The motivation of the followers is in part due to an individualized approach and an adequate level of intellectual stimulation. The focus is on enabling change to occur.[7–9]

Heroic leadership—this approach lives on, but should it?

There is something interesting that happens when we discuss the traits of heroic leaders. If I ask you to imagine one of these old-style leaders, what qualities might you mention?

If I ask you to imagine a 'good strong' leader, what image have you conjured?

Would this 'all-knowing' individual always have all of the answers and be perceived as the expert? Would he or she never show vulnerability or weakness? Could he or she solve all the problems all the time? Would this kind of leader perhaps *tell* people the best way to do things? Would they know what was going on everywhere, all the time? Might they feel responsible for everyone's performance? Would they try to be in control of everything?

I want you to read the last paragraph again but this time, consider the following questions at the same time.

Which of those traits might appeal to you if you are the leader? And why?

And read it one more time asking different questions.

Which of those traits might appeal to you if you are a follower? And why?

Why might heroic leadership appeal and what is the potential downside?

It might be comforting to think that you have control over everything and that you can keep a close eye on the quality of what everyone is doing.

I wonder though how realistic it is to be all things to all people? What if the workload increases? What if the complexity increases? Is it best to have all of the eggs in one basket? What if the leader is off sick or goes under a metaphorical bus?

What about speed and efficiency?

It might be quicker in the short term to simply give people the answers they are looking for or to do their work for them as then at least you can 'make sure it is done properly'!

But, if you never delegate the task or teach anyone else how to achieve it, you will always have to do it yourself. If you allow your staff to be slow and imperfect at first as they learn, but you trust them to develop, they can move up the learning curve and gradually become competent. Once they can achieve the task independently they no longer need to be supervised. This not only makes them feel like they have achieved something and that they are trusted to work on their own, it frees up the time of the leader to be doing something else. Multiple processes can then be running simultaneously which is far more effective in any given situation.

An alternative view—post-heroic leadership

If we unpick this rather unrealistic view of the controlling, all-knowing leader, perhaps we can replace it with something more effective?

Have a look at Table 6.1 for a comparison of heroic and post-heroic attributes and behaviours. As you read the lists be honest with yourself about where you currently sit.

Table 6.1 Heroic versus post-heroic

Heroic	Post-heroic
Has all of the answers	Admits what they don't know, but knows who will know or whether it is possible to know the answer
Is the expert	Consults with experts, including using the different expertise within the team Uses a strengths-based approach to play to the individual team members' strengths
Solves people's problems and tells them what to do, gives advice	Coaches and facilitates, encourages them to find their own answers, challenges dependency
Knows what is going on everywhere, all of the time	Shares responsibility
Is personally responsible for everyone and everything and the performance	Advocates, supports, and develops Empowers Encourages commitment Consults for better solutions
Is in control of everything	Collaborates, enables, delegates Understands that control is not possible anyway
Shows no weakness or vulnerability	Remains authentic Confident enough to be able to show vulnerability and humility

If we consider the two columns, where are you now? How might you wish to alter your thoughts or behaviours? What might you need to do to help you achieve this? What area will you start with?

A modern take on trait theory: Goffee

Goffee[10] revisited the idea that there must be commonalities among successful leaders.

1. From the trait theories, Goffee focused on weaknesses and differences. He did not find common weaknesses but did find that all the exceptional leaders were willing to expose some of their own flaws.

   This fits with the post-heroic style of admitting imperfections and vulnerability. However, confessing to flaws is a balancing act and we will revisit this (an accountant might be best not to admit to being useless with figures).

This fits with the hierarchy of 15 degrees that we have already been promoting (see Level One, p. 60). Admitting vulnerability fits with reducing the steepness of the hierarchy.

2. Goffee found that exceptional leaders were happy to be different. They played to these differences and used their uniqueness as a strength. Goffee asks the question, 'why should anyone be led by you?' Examining your own unique strengths and being in touch with what makes you 'you' might be useful in answering this question yourself.

   In human factors terms we would think of this as being self-aware.

3. From the style theories, Goffee noticed something called 'tough empathy' in the way that the leaders interact with their followers.

   I think this also fits with the human-factors approach of 15 degrees of hierarchy. It is good to be approachable and understanding but not so approachable that the hierarchy is flattened to zero or you lose the role of ultimate decision maker.

4. If we are going to be able to adapt ourselves to different situations, first of all we have to be aware that the situation *has* changed. This requires being a good 'sensor' or being very intuitive, having a combination of self-awareness, situational awareness, and team awareness (the H of SHEEP). It links to the Goleman[4] approach that was discussed in Level One—an emotional intelligence approach to leadership. It fits with an approach of matching a style to a situation but of course first of all you have to be aware of the situation!

Leading with authenticity: George

Bill George[11] confirms the good news: we don't all have to lead in a certain way, we can be true to ourselves; that is, be authentic. George searched for common traits and styles and again came up wanting, but he and his team did discover that there was some common ground shared by all leaders.

The common ground was not life events that fell into themes but instead something about the learning that took place with regards to life events. The great leaders that they studied took responsibility for their own development and didn't expect it to be handed to them on a plate.

So, what big events in your life have shaped you and made you who you are? How did you respond to challenges? What are your core values? How did they develop? Consider Exercise 6.2.

Exercise 6.2 What made you who you are as a leader?

You will need pen and paper or the modern equivalent again.

I want you to draw a straight line across the paper or screen. I want you to divide the line to represent sections of your life in a way that lets you create a timeline.

I want you to think about *who* and *what* have influenced who you are as a leader.

I want you to mark these along the line.

What events have you lived through that changed you or strengthened you, after you had emerged from them? Where do they fit on the line? How have they made you who you are?

What have been the biggest challenges that you have faced? What did you learn from them?

What are you most proud of? How did you achieve that?

Who do you admire? What is it about them that you admire?

Have you come across people who you have vowed *not* to be like? What qualities did they have? Have you successfully kept those traits away?

Have you considered your parents, your school teachers, and your role models, past and present? Who else ended up on the list? Are there any surprises?

Put all of these factors onto your line. How might these things have a positive influence on you? Are there any aspects of yourself that you need to let go of?

The authentic leaders were capable of *reflecting*. They were capable of exploring their own reactions to events. They could reframe the events and look at how they sat with their core values. They were in fact, very in touch with their core values and also what George calls their 'intrinsic motivation'.

I think of intrinsic motivation in terms of 'what floats your boat?' It is fuelled by your life story and the subsequent value system that you have developed over time. It might stem from a desire to develop or help people, change the world or take on social causes. I admit to hoping that if you are in healthcare that people might feature somewhere on your list.

Other people may be motivated by external influences such as power, money, or status.

What drives you? Where do those drives come from? Are your motivations fulfilled in your current role?

The key is self-awareness, which fits in with Goleman's[4] emotional intelligence approach and also with the human-factors approach that we have been encouraging. This time the awareness is about 'what drives or motivates you'. If your external and internal influences can be aligned and somehow balanced with the desires you hold for your home life, you will be happier and be able to lead authentically.

Are you the same 'you' at work, at home, and with your friends? If not, which is the 'real', most authentic you, and how can bring the other spheres of your life more in line with this? Are you expected to behave differently in different settings? Do you wear different 'hats'?

I think we are genuinely lucky in healthcare that our roles involve doing something meaningful. We are all here to help people, however distant you may be from direct patient care. As a personal confession, I would find it far harder to lead if we made widgets, although my sister works for a famous chocolate company and that might have some advantages!

The other common ground discovered among authentic leaders was that they had a great support network. This was usually from a variety of sources including home life, friends, mentors, and their team.

Who do you consider to be in your support network? How do they help you? In what different circumstances would you lean on different people or seek their advice? How do their core values mesh with your own?

The final common theme that George identified was an ability to empower others to lead.

How do you personally empower others? Who was the last person that you might have empowered? If you can't think of anyone, what action might you need to take?

This encourages me to think about what leadership actually involves. The model we are starting to develop is not just of someone in a management role that has leadership written into his or her job description; instead it is something rather different. The picture of leadership that we are starting to build does not define a leader according to where he or she sits in the management structure of the organization. The idea is that anyone throughout the organization can lead or show leadership. The trendy term at the time of writing is 'distributive' leadership. The term might also be applied when the leadership is shared within a team.

Management versus leadership

There are some who will be both managing *and* leading and they may wonder why we are taking the time to differentiate between these two types of skill sets and behaviours. If you are one of these people I would like you to think about which aspects of your role you might wish to delegate—how might you encourage members of your team to take the lead on different tasks? It might also help you to know where your personal strengths might lie so that you can optimize those strengths.

For those of you who currently do not wear a formal managerial hat, I hope to convince you that leadership is relevant to and a possible role for everyone (Box 6.1).

Box 6.1 Soap-box moment

For me, success for the health service would be when staff members no longer feel that they have to ask permission to take initiative, no matter what their grade or position. No matter who the staff were they would answer the phone if it was near them and ringing and would attempt to find an answer; everyone would help a person looking lost in a corridor; everyone would both listen and apologize on behalf of the organization if we are running late and found someone looking distressed; everyone would help resolve car-parking problems; everyone would notice that one of the team hasn't had a break and would cover their work for them so they could grab a bite to eat. There are pockets of these behaviours across the NHS. I have seen them. If we can empower everyone to make them feel we are truly all in this together, banging the same drum, that is what success would constitute for me. If we have aligned people to care, to take the initiative, and to deliver a safe and effective patient-centred service, that would be the result of great leadership.

Climbing down from the soap box—apologies for the passionate outburst!

Kotter[12] suggests that management produces order and consistency. He describes planning, budgeting, staffing, organizing, controlling, and problem solving as management activities.

He suggests that leadership, on the other hand, focuses on producing change and movement. Leadership activities include vision building, strategy, aligning people, communicating, motivating, and inspiring.

Of course, in a successful organization all of these activities ought to be taking place, but they do not have to be the responsibility of just one individual.

Rittel and Webber[13] approach the issue from another direction. They looked at the problems or challenges we face, whether they were complicated but resolvable and had probably been faced before, in which case they were classified as *tame* problems that are suitable for a *managerial* solution. The manager would provide the *processes* that in turn provide the solution. However, if the problem was novel, complex, and difficult to understand, difficult to classify, difficult to be clear about, so that it was not resolvable through the usual solution-focused processes, the problem was classed as a *wicked* problem. Wicked problems require leadership and collective effort. There are no black-and-white answers, (perhaps no answers at all) and no definitive right and wrong. Grint[14–18] suggests that in this setting, the key is to ask the right questions. I would suggest that this questioning approach may be harnessed to result in creative decision making or option generation and choice. There may not be an end to the problem.

Grint discusses a third category of problem, the *crisis*, which he suggests invites a *commander* or authoritarian approach. (I believe the background for this approach lies in military contexts rather than in healthcare.)

Grint suggests that the *commander* seeks an *answer*, the *manager* a *process*, and the *leader* a *question*. He is not inferring that a problem ever fits neatly into one of these categories, or that there is a perfect way to deal with each category.

He goes on to suggest that we can be guilty of defining the problem in the way we would like to deal with it. For example, if we favour a commander-type approach, we may interpret problems as a crisis. (If you want to read more, this longer article[18] allows you to explore complex social models in more depth).

I think it is vital that even in a crisis setting in healthcare we encourage input from the team and don't let the hierarchy steepen towards a commander-type approach. Whilst I agree that we face time-pressured decision making, the shared mental model and shared decision making can help to prevent fixation error, assumption, bias, and the experience of many people can result in better solutions. In a life-threatening complex emergency in healthcare, we encourage the leader to stand back and take a hands-off approach (where staffing numbers allow). I would expect our leader to take the 'big picture' or balcony view. I encourage him or her to put his or her hands in pockets in an attempt to stop 'doing', and instead hope that he or she will be 'watching' and 'listening' avidly. I don't agree they should be enforcing a steep hierarchy in their team nor should they be making unilateral, autocratic decisions. I would expect this leader to be gathering ideas and encouraging option generation from the team.

There are clinical parallels for the tame and wicked problems. If the emergency department is filling up rapidly and there are people in the corridors waiting for beds and ambulances starting to queue outside, you would want your senior decision makers to be involved. This is complex; there is not a single-point solution to this problem. Whilst the problem may have occurred before, the solution each time will be unique because of the enormous number of variables that must be taken into account.

For a 'routine' cardiac arrest, there is a team and a rule-based approach and despite the fact that it is an emergency, it need not be a crisis. It can be well run, organized, and rehearsed. It can be efficiently undertaken without consultant input. It is a 'tame' problem for the NHS staff in this case, but a crisis for the patient concerned. Assuming the patient survives, he or she may need to address lifestyle issues such as diet, exercise, and smoking habits that may well constitute a very wicked problem for them.

The cardiac arrests that I would choose to attend as a consultant were the ones that were unusual. The cardiac arrest in the reception area (which is not close to a clinical area), the one in the car park, or half-way up a corridor, or somewhere that was isolated such as a Portakabin®. In these much more unusual settings, few people have dealt with that problem before. It is trickier to sort out new logistics in an unfamiliar environment. This is where senior decision makers come in to their own. It is the unfamiliar environment that converts the 'tame' problem into a 'wicked' problem. It may not be possible to deliver the treatment as per the protocol because the kit won't be present. It may be that the equipment won't fit into the space where the patient currently lies following the collapse. It may be that there is a 'crowd-control' problem with lots of people watching and the patient's dignity is in need of preserving. Do we move the kit or the patient? When and how and with whom and with what? We are trying to solve all of these problems as well as follow the guidelines for the cardiac arrest. This is when it becomes a 'wicked' problem. You could, however, argue that it is possible to resolve these issues relatively easily and you will be able to find solutions to these, even if they are not perfect. Perhaps the really wicked problem lies, as we already suggested, with the patient who will have to cope with lifestyle changes (see Figure 6.1).

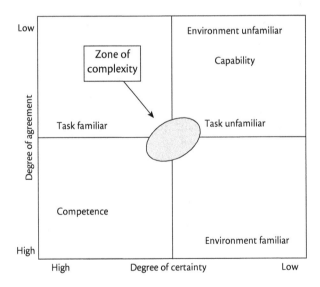

Figure 6.1 Competence and capability in complex adaptive systems.
Reproduced with permission from Fraser S and Greenhalgh T, Coping with complexity: educating for capability, *British Medical Journal*, Volume 323, Issue 7316, pp. 799–803, Copyright © 2001.

Some contemporary ideas about leadership

The imperfect leader: Ancona

Ancona[19] suggests that in reality no leader ticks all of the leadership boxes. She identifies four categories that she has found to represent the kind of leadership that organizations need, but she would not expect to find all of those qualities within one individual. Reassuringly, she encourages leaders to identify and then play to their strengths, whilst filling the gaps with team members who have the complementary skills.

Sense making

This style of leader is quick to grasp how an organization (or department) works and within what context, the way this changes and how others might understand it. It ties in with emotional intelligence, and with situational awareness. Leadership is a continuous process forged from a combination of 'observations, data, experiences, conversations, and analyses'.[19]

Relating

Leaders in this category are good at building trusting relationships and networks. This is the people section. It fits with the 'H' of SHEEP and with Lencioni's[20] triangle, the first step of which is trust. Ancona[19] suggests there are three components within this domain: *advocacy*, *inquiry*, and *connecting*. The *advocacy* component comprises simply explaining one's own view. It also involves explaining *why* you hold that view. *Inquiry* involves asking questions and then listening attentively so that you understand the thoughts and feelings of the other party. The *connecting* domain is the vital activity of networking. By eliciting views from a range of sources and encouraging questions from these, the leader will get the widest possible input into whatever conundrum presents itself.

Visioning

This is a future-focused technique. It involves creating imagery that is perceived as realistic and appealing. It is about the leader creating a shared understanding among staff of this future state and a shared desire to achieve it. It has nothing to do with writing a motto on a wall! It has everything to do with enthusiasm, great communication skills, motivation, generating excitement, and good organizational information flow. It involves the use of images, metaphors, and storytelling that can translate complex issues into something easy to grasp and desire.

Inventing

This leadership skill involves creativity. It is also about action. By finding new ways of doing things the steps to achieve a new future are translated into actions. This not only involves generating new ideas but also new ways of working together. It will also involve stopping doing some of the things we have usually done.

Ancona's[19] approach fits in nicely with a human-factors approach. We all make mistakes; we are allowed to be less than perfect. We do not have to strive to house all of those qualities in just one person; they can be shared across our team.

Adaptive leadership: Heifetz

Heifetz presents a very challenging perspective on leadership that comprises a way of thinking about the difficult things organizations face (and usually avoid) than a simple list of dos and dont's.[21] Some of his useful ideas include:

Balcony and the dance floor

We have already explored the concept of the balcony and the dance floor in Level One and earlier in this book. It is a concept that I find very useful when teaching the concept of self-awareness. Whether it is possible to teach self-awareness itself is a completely different question. This is the first of six useful ideas from Heifetz.[21]

Identify your adaptive challenges

'Adaptive challenges can only be addressed through changes in people's priorities, beliefs, habits, and loyalties. Making progress requires going beyond authoritative expertise to mobilize discovery, shedding certain entrenched ways, tolerating losses, and generating new capacity to thrive anew' (Heifetz et al.).[22]

This epitomizes for me what we are trying to achieve with human-factors training. We need to move away from the emphasis on teaching knowledge and technical skills in isolation and instead blend them with the relevant non-technical skills. We need to improve communication skills, challenge ingrained hierarchies, generate a culture driven by continuous learning, and take a new approach to error awareness and improving safety.

When we face adaptive challenges we need to stop trying to tackle them with technical solutions or, worse still, avoid them altogether.

Regulate distress

Heifetz[21] suggests that by controlling the rate of change it is possible to strike a balance between asking tough questions and maintaining momentum whilst providing clear direction and communicating key issues and values. Some initiatives may need to cease in order to allow others to start, and this will help keep the process of change from becoming overwhelming. Anxiety levels need to be managed—too much change all at once and people panic, but too little and momentum can be lost; there's no energy or reason to change things or act or react differently.

Maintain disciplined attention

If a conflict arises don't deal with it superficially or allow denial of its existence. Unpick the problem and try to get to the heart of the issue. Keep everyone focused on the difficult adaptive challenges; don't let them get distracted by the easier technical or practical ones. Encourage a collaborative approach to problem solving.

Give the work back to the employees

We have already used the word 'empower' at regular intervals. Empowering involves increasing the self-confidence of others and reducing their dependency on those higher up the hierarchy. The emphasis here is on supporting and challenging people rather than controlling them. This involves encouraging risk taking but also being ready to back people up if they make an error. Heifetz[21] takes this much further and proposes taking the really difficult challenges (changing ways of working, culture shifts, attitude and belief changes) and demanding that people engage with these instead of avoiding them or pushing these 'up' to senior managers. This is difficult but crucial work for the leader. There is shared responsibility across the team (see Example 6.1) and also across the organization.

Example 6.1 A theatre team

I want you to consider a fictitious surgeon and his theatre team. He is frustrated because they have worked together for a number of years and yet there are some recurring errors with the set-up of the theatre. There is regularly a problem with the way the suction is attached and some of the instruments are missing from the sets. The team seems to think that it is his responsibility to sort these things out. Team members view the recurring small errors as unimportant. The surgeon finds the omissions irritating. It interrupts his thought process at a vital point in the operation to have to remind the team about the missing suction and equipment. He finds it hard to concentrate on the next steps and is worried that he will make a mistake.

What should he do?

What he currently does is to talk about it in the debrief at the end of the list and ask that it improves next time. Or occasionally he gets cross with everyone. The theatre team members are apologetic and they promise they will remember but no improvement has occurred over several years.

Heifetz[21] encourages us to give the responsibility for solving the problem to the team. He describes how they might not want to take on the responsibility and how they might try to give it back.

The required conversation might proceed as follows:

(Starting with an SBIC approach.)

'I am finding the recurring errors with the suction and missing equipment very frustrating. It interrupts my concentration at an important part of the procedure. How are we going to change this?'

Now he waits and uses silence. He sits and says nothing else. If after several minutes no ideas are forthcoming, he might add.

'I need to know how we are going to stop this from recurring.'

Waits again. He does not offer any solutions of his own nor make suggestions.

Once the ideas start it may be possible to switch into a coaching style.

'What else might help?'

'How will that work?'

'Who is going to do that bit?'

'What if they aren't here?'

'When will it start?'

'How likely is it to succeed on a scale of 1 to 10?'

'What would change that to a 10?'

The idea is to create shared ownership of the problem and shared responsibility.

Protect leadership voices from below

Heifetz[21] encourages us all to speak up if we can see a problem. It doesn't matter where you consider yourself to be in the hierarchy, have the assertiveness to voice your concerns. We need to generate a workplace culture that will make this acceptable, where it is better to say something and be wrong than to have kept quiet and be right (I knew that was going to happen!). This is true not only from a safety perspective but it also encourages creative solutions. Even if some new ideas generated won't work, we ought to encourage this kind of thinking. Without new ideas, we will stagnate and fail to make progress. We need to make it safe and totally acceptable to put ideas forward. I often hear about a 'fear of speaking up in case I looked stupid'. It is this that we have to overcome; we need to work on building up this psychological safety within the culture of our organization.

The other concept that Heifetz[21] introduces is the concept of leadership as learning. As an educator this concept excites me. I love to learn and I love to help others to learn.

The question he encourages us to ask is, '*who needs to learn what in order to develop, understand, commit to, and implement the strategy?*'

Holding that question in your head, I would like you to consider again what I have said previously, which I will repeat here:

We need to move away from the emphasis on teaching knowledge and technical skills in isolation and instead blend them with the relevant non-technical skills. We need to improve communication skills, challenge ingrained hierarchies, generate a culture of continuous learning, and take a new approach to error awareness and improving safety.

If we are to achieve these adaptive challenges, it cannot be the sole remit of the board or the executive to lead these changes. It will need leadership from below and across the organization. This will require truly distributive leadership where we all commit to bringing these changes into existence.

What role will you play?

If we try to bring all of these thoughts on leadership together and combine it with a human-factors approach, what might the end results be?

Box 6.2 offers a glimpse of what happens if we adapt the generic non-technical skills tool to an issue that is non-clinical and leadership orientated.

Box 6.2

Team

- Leadership skills
  - Authenticity
  - Admit to vulnerability

- Show humility
- Dare to be different
- Collaborates, enables, delegates
- Challenges dependency
- Coaches, facilitates
- Protects voices from below
- Tough empathy
- 'Followership' skills
  - Assertiveness
  - Strengths-based approach
  - Keep the leader grounded
- Team building and maintaining
  - Hierarchy management
  - Clear and appropriate role allocation
  - Motivation
  - Gives the work back to the team
  - Willing to adapt to unfamiliar roles and ways of working
  - Consideration and support of others
  - Advocacy with inquiry
  - Networking
- Conflict solving
  - Balances the tension between progress and conflict
  - Unpick what is underlying the conflict, delve deeper

Decision making

- Problem definition and diagnosis
  - Commentating
  - Generating shared mental model
  - Avoiding biases

- Option generation
  - Encouraging team input
  - Avoiding fixation error
  - Encouraging creativity for new ways of working and novel ideas
- Risk assessment and option selection
  - Shared decision making
- Regular review of decision as new information emerges
  - Shared responsibility

Tasks

- Providing and maintaining standards
  - Attention to detail
- Workload management
  - Identify adaptive challenges
  - Adapt to new tasks
  - Distraction management
  - Prioritization of tasks
  - Control the rate of change of the tasks
  - Shared responsibility for task completion and quality

Awareness—situational

- Awareness of the systems
- Awareness of the environment in which the organization/department sits
- Sensing the situation
- Awareness of time
- Ability to plan ahead

Awareness—self

- Stress, fatigue, cognitive workload, time pressure
- Call for help if appropriate
  - Know your own limitations
  - Know when to consult

- Balcony and dance floor
- Swan
- Self-regulation

Information management

- Gathering of information
- Sharing of information
- Visioning
  - Use of imagery, metaphors, and storytelling
  - Setting direction
- Listening, non-verbal and verbal communication
- Ask the tough questions
- Unpick divisive issues
- Social skills

Key points (up to and including Chapter 6)

- Situational awareness can be considered as having three components:
  - perception (*what?*),
  - comprehension (*so what?*), and
  - predicting future state (*what next?*).
- We make sense of what we have perceived so that it becomes a working mental model.
- When working in a team it is important that the *mental model* is shared with, and shared by, the team members.
- Remember that *commentating* is a skill where we talk our thoughts aloud. This not only slows our thinking down and makes it more deliberate, it also helps to control our stress levels and it helps others to understand what we thinking. The latter links to generating a shared mental model.
- This shared mental model builds towards a team situational assessment or problem definition.

- Barriers to perception and comprehension include:

  - high workload,

  - time pressure,

  - perceived high risk,

  - stress,

  - fatigue,

  - biases (including expectation, confirmation and environmental), and

  - task fixation.

- When building our mental model problems can arise due to:

  - missed cues,

  - misinterpreting cues, or

  - choosing to ignore cues,

  - incorrect risk assessment,

  - poor time judgement, or

  - a failure to update our mental model either when new information becomes available or when conditions change.

- It can be useful to do a quick run through of **SHEEP** to help with situational awareness.

  - S—which guideline/SOP are we using? Do we have all of the information we need?

  - H—who is doing what? How is that working? Is someone time keeping?

  - E—are we in the best place for what confronts us?

  - E—do we have all the kit that we need?

  - P—how full is my bucket? Where is my focus?

- Once we have completed our situational assessment or problem definition we move to, '*what are we going to do about it?*'

- There are four main types of decision-making process:

  - *recognition-primed or intuitive,*

  - *rule-based,*

* ◆ *option generation*, and

* ◆ *creative*

◆ How we decide which method suits the situation depends on time pressure, risk, and the novelty of the situation.

◆ The rule-based approach for emergencies exists to make life easier for us.

◆ When we have more time we can use an option-generation model such as DECIDE.

◆ Making a decision is only the first step in a cycle. We should then continuously monitor that treatment or plan and review it. This is especially true in the light of new information.

◆ It is vital to update our mental model with new information.

◆ Please guard against the *assumption* that the diagnosis is definitely correct.

◆ We need to spend more time reviewing how we are making our decisions so that we can improve this skill.

◆ Conflict can be considered as an **unmet need**.

◆ Conflict can be classed as substantive or personal.

◆ Substantive conflict has a place in change or in moving things forward. It isn't always negative.

◆ It is worth understanding the conflict triangle: people—who is fighting and where are the clashes, process—how does the conflict manifest itself, and the underlying problem—what are they fighting about?

◆ When personal conflict occurs, in understanding people it is worth unpicking why it has occurred and trying to understand it in terms of MBTI styles, preferred learning styles (Honey and Mumford), and preferred team roles (Belbin).

◆ When helping to resolve conflict some basic tools are useful; listening skills, perfecting your 'interested', open questioning, and an understanding of eye contact, posture, stillness, and the importance of planning the environment.

◆ The next important skill is mastering your 'attention'. Improvement with this skill can be helped with mindfulness.

◆ Other skills that are useful to develop in these settings are self-awareness, self-management, and the management of your own value and belief system.

- Other skills to acquire include summarizing, reflecting back, positive reframing, hypothesis, pre-framing, prompts, clarifying questions, and appreciative enquiry.

- A mediator may be necessary and very helpful in resolving some conflicts.

- Some of the additional tools a mediator may use include 'normalizing', 'mutualizing', past-to-future state, concatenation, and a skilful use of the positive reframe.

- Hierarchy management has an important role in conflict resolution.

- The graded assertiveness tool CUSS can be useful when you need to highlight a concern but don't know quite how to tackle the subject. It stands for Concern, Unsure, Safety, and Stop.

- Once conflict has been resolved, there needs to be some time invested in developing the team.

- Coaching has a role to play in both individual and team development.

- A commonly used approach in coaching is TGROW: Topic, Goal, Reality, Options, and Will/Wrap up.

- When considering team development it can be helpful to use Hawkins' approach: CLEAR (contracting, listening, exploring, action, and review).

- Hawkins suggests the team look at external fit, internal focus, how they will work together, and who else will the team work with.

- Lencione suggests there are five main causes of a dysfunctional team:
  - absence of trust,
  - fear of conflict,
  - lack of commitment,
  - avoidance of accountability, and
  - inattention to results.

- Debriefing helps us achieve double-loop learning.

- Honey and Mumford describe four preferred learning styles: activists, pragmatists, theorists, and reflectors.

- We need to cater for all learning styles.

- There are a number of debriefing models to use as a framework. I use the traffic cone method of vent, description, analysis, generalize/apply to real situations.

- Useful techniques include 80:20, open questions, appreciative enquiry, use of silence, summarizing, reflect back, hypothesis, pre-framing, paraphrasing, and 'normalizing'.

- We should all aim for a daily debrief, even if we work on our own: 'what did I learn today?' 'How will that change what I do in the future?'

- After-action review is another simple framework to use.

- My slightly adapted version of the after-action review is:

  - **what did you expect to happen?**

  - **what actually happened?**

  - **what are the differences between these?**

  - **how do you think they came about? Consider SHEEP.**

  - **what have we learned?**

- Modern thoughts on leadership go beyond trait theories and heroic leadership.

- Goffee suggests successful leaders show vulnerability, are happy to be different, demonstrate tough empathy, and are great at reading a situation.

- Kotter[12] suggests that management produces order and consistency. He describes planning, budgeting, staffing, organizing, controlling, and problem solving as management activities.

- Kotter suggests that leadership, on the other hand, focuses on producing change. The parallel activities for leadership are described as vision building, strategy, aligning people, communicating, motivating, and inspiring.

- Ancona advocates sense making, relating, visioning, and inventing but acknowledges that these skills are not necessarily found in one individual and they can be the result of a team effort.

- Heifetz usefully proposes the balcony and the dance floor metaphor, identification of the adaptive challenges, regulating distress, maintaining disciplined attention, leaving responsibility for the adaptive challenges with the whole team, and protecting the voices from below.

- Heifetz encourages us to think of leadership as learning and to ask the question, *'who needs to learn what in order to develop, understand, commit to and implement the strategy?'*

I apologize if your favourite leadership author has not been included in my list. This is a high level overview. As I said at the beginning, there are more textbooks on leadership than there are on medicine and I don't have space to cite them all.

References

1. Lewin K, Heider F, Heider GM. *Principles of Topological Psychology*, 1st edn. New York, NY: McGraw-Hill, 1936.
2. Lewin K. *The Conceptual Representation and the Measurement of Psychological Forces*. Durham, NC: Duke University Press, 1938.
3. Mouton J and Blake R. *The Managerial Grid: The Key to Leadership Excellence*. Houston, TX: Gulf Publishing Co., 1964.
4. Goleman D. What Makes a Leader? *Harvard Business Review* 1998; 76(6): 93–102.
5. French JRP and Raven BH. The Bases of Social Power. In Cartwright D et al. (ed.). *Studies in Social Power*. Ann Arbor: MI: Institute for Social Research, 1959, pp. 150–67.
6. Raven B. The Bases of Power and the Power/Interaction Model of Interpersonal Influence. *Analyses of Social Issues and Public policy* 2008; 8(1): 1–22.
7. Bass BM, Riggio RE. *Transformational Leadership*, 2nd edn. Mahwah, NJ: Lawrence Erlbaum Associates, 2006.
8. Bass BM. The Implications of Transactional and Transformational Leadership for Individual, Team and Organizational Development. In: Pasmore R (ed.). *Research in Organizational Change and Devleopment*. Greenwich: JAI Press, 1990: pp. 231–72.
9. Burns JM. *Leadership*. New York, NY: Harper & Row, 1979.
10. Goffee R, Jones G. *Why Should Anyone be Led by You?: What it Takes to be an Authentic Leader*. Boston, MA: Harvard Business School Press, 2006.
11. George B. Authentic Leadership: Rediscovering the Secrets to Creating Lasting Value. *Warren Bennis Signature Series*, 1st edn. San Francisco, CA: Jossey-Bass, 2003: 1 online resource (xix, L 217 p.).
12. Kotter JP. *John P. Kotter on what Leaders Really Do*. Boston, MA: Harvard Business School Press, 1999.
13. Webber R. Dilemmas in a General Theory of Planning. *Policy Sciences* 1973; 4: 155–69.
14. Grint K. *Leadership: Classical, Contemporary, and Critical Approaches*. Oxford: Oxford University Press, 1997.
15. Grint K. *Leadership: Limits and Possibilities*. Basingstoke: Palgrave Macmillan, 2005.
16. Grint K. *Leadership, Management and Command: Rethinking D-Day*. Basingstoke: Palgrave Macmillan, 2008.
17. Grint K. *Leadership: A Very Short Introduction*. Oxford: Oxford University Press, 2010.
18. Grint K. Problems, Problems, Problems: The Social Construction of Leadership. *Human Relations*, 2005; 58(11): 1467–94.
19. Ancona D, Malone TW, Orlikowski WJ, et al. In Praise of the Incomplete Leader. *Harvard Business Review* 2007; 85(2): 92–100, 56.
20. Lencioni PM. Make Your Values Mean Something. *Harvard Business Review* 2002; 80(7): 113–7, 26.
21. Heifetz R. *Leadership Without Easy Answers*. Cambridge, MA: Belknap Press of Harvard University Press, 1994.
22. Heifetz R, Glashow A, Linsky M. *Practice of Adpative Leadership: Tools and Tactics for Changing Your Organization and The World*. Cambridge, MA: Harvard Business Review Press, 2009.

7

Learning culture

What is wanted is not the will to believe, but the wish to find out, which is its exact opposite.

Bertrand Russell, 1872–1970

British philosopher and mathematician: *Free Thought and Official Propaganda* (1922)

So what is a learning culture?

A learning culture within a department, or potentially within a whole organization, is where continuous improvement becomes the norm. Peter Senge[1,2] has described five components of a learning culture that are adapted here and given a human factors tweak.

Personal mastery

This involves creating an environment for the individual and the organization in which goals for each can be developed, aligned, and realized.

Mental models

Understanding how your mental model and situational awareness will influence your decision making and behaviour is vital.

Shared vision

Generating shared mental models of the future and using shared decision making allows the group to commit to these shared aims. This replaces the old cliché of aligning people to the vision, as they have created the vision themselves rather than having it imposed upon them. This moves us away from the idea of following a 'vision statement' for the organization. It is about first, jointly creating ideas about the future, what will work, decided by the people who will be doing the work. It must fit with the overall direction of the organization but the impetus comes from distributive leadership, not top-down command and control.

Team learning

This component incorporates the idea that the groups' capability (or ability to develop) is greater than the sum of its individual talents. This can be used to develop collective intelligence, emotional intelligence, thinking skills, problem solving, and decision making, grappling with adaptive challenges and technical abilities. It concerns tackling values, beliefs, behaviours, and the drivers for these, together with a keen awareness of collective responsibility.

System thinking

Every team is capable of 'big picture' thinking at both departmental and organizational level. It must understand where it fits into the organizational jigsaw and how changes in the team may affect other parts of the organization.

We will now explore the two terms, *learning* and *culture*, in more detail, and consider in more depth how we might achieve this nirvana of a learning culture where we continuously improve and generate a culture that encourages learning, from both positive and negative events, on a daily basis across the organization.

Culture

Cook and Yanow[3] define culture as, 'A set of values, beliefs and feelings, together with the artefacts of their expression and transmission (such as myths, symbols, metaphors and rituals) that are created, inherited, shared and transmitted within one group of people.'

A more informal definition is 'the way we do things around here'.

There are differences of opinion as to whether culture change is possible at all. I believe it is but I am not deluded enough to think it will happen overnight. Learning to alter our 'values, beliefs and feelings' is quite a challenge. It is rather different from learning how to perform a practical skill! I want to spend some time exploring how we learn.

How do adults learn?

We have already touched on the theory proposed by Honey and Mumford[4] and on double-loop learning[5]. I want to add a little more educational theory here.

In the simplest terms, we learn through a combination of 'doing', 'thinking', 'understanding theory', and 'experimenting'.

There are far fancier ways of describing the processes and I have included Kolb's learning cycle[6] (see Figure 7.1), on which I have superimposed Honey and Mumford's[4] styles and parallel ideas from Gibbs[7] (Figure 7.2) and Grant[8] (Figure 7.3) so that you can explore them in more depth knowing the correct terminology.

There are many ways of thinking about learning styles. I want you to consider whether you prefer visual input (colours, diagrams, pictures, a 'show-me' approach), or auditory input (verbal and other sounds, 'tell me'), or kinaesthetic learning (touching or physically doing something to understand it,) (and no, it isn't 'touch me'! It is 'let me do it').

Which model of learning do you prefer? Why? Do you prefer grand terminology or a simplified approach? What does that tell you about you? Why have I included three models?

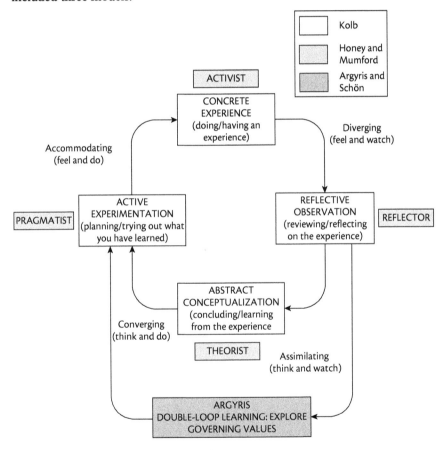

Figure 7.1 Combined learning cycle.

Source: data from Kolb DA, *Experiential learning: experience as the source of learning and development.* Englewood Cliffs, NJ: Prentice Hall, 1984; Honey P and Mumford A, *The learning Styles Questionnaire: 80-item version.* Maidenhead: Peter Honey Publications, 2006; Argyris C and Schön DA, *Theory in practice: increasing professional effectiveness.* San Francisco, CA: Jossey-Bass, 1974.

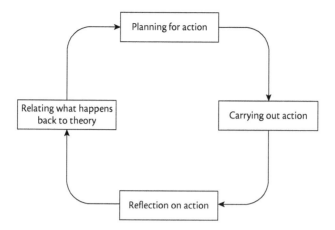

Figure 7.2 Gibbs' learning cycle.

Reproduced with permission from Gibbs G, *Learning by Doing: a guide to teaching and learning methods*. Oxford: Oxford Centre for Staff and Learning Development, Oxford Brookes University, 1988. Copyright © 1988 Oxford Brookes University.

The 'doing' bit seems to be important to adult learners. We know that experiential learning, learning by doing, is a powerful adult learning tool.[9]

There are a couple of other things I want you to consider.

How do you know what you know?

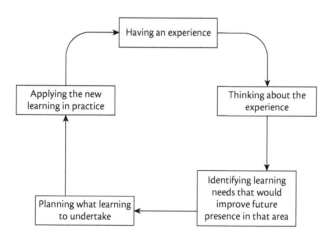

Figure 7.3 Grant's learning cycle.

Source: data from Grant J and Marsden P. *Training senior house officers by service based training*. Joint Conference for Education in Medicine. London, 1992. Also published in *British Medical Journal* 1989;299:1263–68.

Almost more importantly, how do you know what you do not know? This links to self-awareness. We need to know when we are at the limits of our knowledge base and perhaps our skills. We need to know when we are out of our depth and when we should call for help. It is worth exploring the concept of your Johari[10] window in this context (see Figure 7.4).

Abraham Maslow is usually credited with a model of learning that suggests we start with unconscious incompetence. He suggests that we progress through conscious incompetence to conscious competence and finally to unconscious competence.

Can you think of an example of a knowledge area or skill you possess that fits into each of those levels? Cooking a chocolate fondant versus boiling an egg? Doing a new-born baby check? Riding a bicycle versus driving a high performance car? Anaesthetizing for varicose vein removal or a ruptured aortic aneurysm repair? Delivering a baby? GCSE maths? Human factors? Photography? Computing? Leadership?

Whilst we of course want our staff to be given a good education, we also want them to be able to learn on the job, every day, by just making small stepwise improvements in the way they do things.

As we are dealing exclusively with adult learners, they will have a preference in the way that they like to learn. This will be influenced by personality preferences, past experience, prior knowledge, personal values, beliefs, assumptions, and expectations.

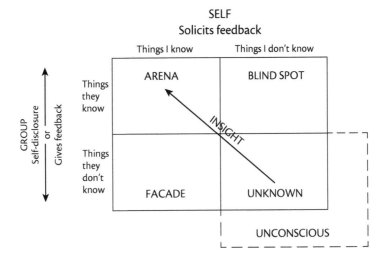

Figure 7.4 The Johari window.

Reproduced with permission from Luft J. *Group Processes: an introduction to group dynamics*. 3rd edn. Mountain View, CA: Mayfield Publishing. Copyright © 1984 McGraw-Hill, Inc.

Whether we choose to learn depends partly on our motivation.

In the context of an educational course, I observe a difference in the motivational levels between those who chose to attend the course compared with those who were 'sent'.

> Is what we are learning an essential qualification for our role (e.g. an advanced life-support course)?

> If we gain this qualification, might it help us get a promotion?

> What about the motivation for continuous improvement? Where does that come from?

> How will you take your team with you so that they just want to improve every day too? Who might already be working in that manner on your team? Who will be quick to follow? Who will present more of a challenge? How will you tackle that?

Some of how we learn on the job is by done as apprentices. This can be referred to as social learning. We learn by observing others, following them as role models, watching and copying their behaviour and techniques. Some of this learning is unconscious and some more conscious. (I like the way A does that but I'll mix that with how B does that bit. I'll avoid what C does!) This is why who we select as role models is so important!

What are you role modelling?

Bloom's taxonomy[11–14] divides the classic triad of knowledge, skills, and attitudes into three domains: cognitive, psychomotor, and affective. It breaks down learning into stages for each domain. The stages of the cognitive domain[11] are: recalling data, understanding, applying or using it, analysing it, synthesizing it, and evaluating it. For the psychomotor domain these stages comprise: imitation, manipulation under instruction, develop precision, articulation (combining and integrating skills), and naturalization (becoming an expert). For the affective domain[13] they are: receiving (gaining awareness), responding (reacting), valuing (understanding and acting), organizing one's personal value system, and internalizing one's value system (adopting behaviour). (There are useful thoughts on measurement and assessment at the various stages presented within Bloom's taxonomy.)

In which of these domains do you currently teach? Are you more comfortable with some than others? Which do you find most challenging?

Traditionally in healthcare we have focused, almost entirely, on knowledge and skill transfer. It is time to tackle the affective domain more robustly! How might you tackle this with your team or trainees or students? Which values or behaviours might you wish to tackle? How might you go about the first step of raising awareness?

Kirkpatrick's theory[15] helps us to explore how to assess the impact of education and training. Kirkpatrick's model is usually displayed as a pyramid with the simplest layer at the bottom and the most complex at the top. The levels from basic to complex are:

1. Reaction: what did participants actually think (or feel) about the training? This is the equivalent of filling in what I colloquially refer to as a 'happy sheet' at the end of the training episode.

2. Learning: can you demonstrate an increase in knowledge or skill or a change in attitude or behaviour? For example, use a before-and-after questionnaire that demonstrates a difference between knowledge prior to and after the training.

3. Behaviour: can you demonstrate that the training led to a behavioural change when the person returns to his or her normal job? Try assessment 3/6/12 months after the course looking for changes.

4. Outcomes/results: can you demonstrate a change in patient outcome or some other results (e.g. a decrease in error rate, higher morale, reduced waste, improved patient experience, improved staff retention, a decrease in complaints)?

When planning an educational intervention you should start with these level four results in mind.

Learning: An alternative viewpoint to consider

I want to reiterate that leadership can be thought of as learning.

Let's return to the complex adaptive challenges; not the easy technical challenges that we face but instead some of the 'stuff' that induces us to adopt an ostrich-type approach, the type of thing that you might have on your 'too-hard' pile.

Consider some challenges where there is no easy answer to be found. If, when you read the following examples, you find yourself thinking, 'that's easy', stop for a moment. You may be missing some of the layers of complexity. Consider those layers.

◆ Consider a complex interpersonal problem within a department. For example, X, and Y, and Z have a private practice agreement that gives them power over C. There is a problem with Y in the NHS but C doesn't want to say anything. D is a new consultant and doesn't want to take sides. There is a change that the department needs to implement. D has been made responsible tasked with bringing in the change but feels worried that he does not have the seniority to do so as he is the junior consultant colleague.

◆ Think about a practice of GPs who are partners and some salaried GPs who are not. There is a disparity between the number of clinics/number of patients being seen by one partner, which is far fewer than the others. There are differences in the amount of leave each GP can take.

◆ What about a situation where entrenched processes and behaviours are outmoded but no-one is brave enough to try to change them? Think of a governance meeting where 40 people are supposed to attend where nothing is ever decided and no actions result. The arguments are cyclical and the behaviours are often aggressive and intimidating, with an attitude of 'whoever shouts the loudest wins'.

◆ Perhaps savings have to be made but some departments are being more cooperative than others. Some departments are saying they simply cannot cost cut and are still ordering new equipment without considering the effect on other areas. Perhaps these departments traditionally bring in a large amount income and so argue that they should not be subject to the same cuts as other departments. Perhaps they are also tougher at negotiating when the leads have to put forward their ideas. This is perceived as unfair by other departments and is causing unrest.

◆ There has been a difference between the ways different staff groups were treated following an error. The different professional groups have taken an entirely different approach from one another. One group used a learning conversation and explored the topic. The other group had a knee-jerk response and suspended the person they believed made the error until there was an investigation. There is now complete disharmony between the multi-professional members of the team. They are refusing to engage in MDTs until the disciplinary process has been stopped.

How would you help people to explore values, attitudes, behaviours, and learning whilst encouraging creative thinking and leaving shared responsibility for the problem solving with those with the problem?

People who think they can wave a magic wand and produce culture change do not fully understand the complexity of the issues we face.

Capability

The *Oxford English Dictionary* definition of capability is '*the power or ability to do something*' (*Oxford English Dictionary*, 2011). In our setting we are looking at capability as the ability to adapt to change, to acquire new knowledge, skills, and behaviours, and to generate continuous improvement.

Learning that develops capability takes place when we engage with something uncertain and unfamiliar. We are forced to shift perspectives, question assumptions, and re-examine expectations. By applying existing knowledge and competencies in a novel way we can adapt to new situations (see Figure 6.1).

Current culture

I do not believe that the culture is uniform across the NHS. I notice a massive difference of culture even within one hospital and even within a department in the hospital depending on who is 'on'.

However, if we use an incredibly broad brush-stroke we can compare and contrast where some micro-cultures might be and where we might want to be (see Table 7.1). As you read through the Table, I want you to consider things from three perspectives: you, your department, and your executive team or equivalent.

Table 7.1 Target-driven versus learning culture

Target-driven culture	Learning culture
Focus on targets	Focus on improvement Focus on staff development
Listen to the patient (especially the friends and family 'test'. Hit the target)	Learn from the patient
Hit the numbers	See beyond the numbers
Fix the root cause, add in another layer of safety, tick a box	Double-loop learning, multiple causes of errors explored, a deep understanding of the behaviours and values that underlie the errors
Execute the plan	Monitor and re-evaluate the plan, continuous improvement of the plan
Fix the weaknesses, big stick	Play to the strengths Raise morale Motivated, happy staff
Top down	Distributive leadership
'Thou must be caring and show empathy!'	Free staff up from non-critical tasks to allow them to give the care they would like to deliver; they are naturally caring

(continued)

206

Table 7.1 Target-driven versus learning culture *(continued)*

Target-driven culture	Learning culture
Recruit entirely based on expertise	Recruit for values in addition to expertise
Do your job and get it done now	Do your job Improve on the current systems and processes that affect your job and how you perform it
Pace-setting leadership style predominates	Range of leadership styles used, people are encouraged to take initiative, encourage creative thinking
Steep hierarchy	15 degrees of hierarchy This enables people of all levels to ask questions
Senior leaders are task or target focused	Role modelling of senior leaders spending time talking about learning and considering values, beliefs, attitudes, and behaviours
Appraisal used as a box-ticking exercise; we have hit the target for the number of appraisals	Appraisal as a developmental tool, a learning conversation, including a focus on what has been learned. The staff feel valued, supported, appropriately challenged, and praised
Education, other than mandatory training, is a luxury and is not a priority	Education is vital if we are to improve and needs to be adequately resourced and prioritized, and staff must be freed up so that we can educate them
Errors only handled with single-loop learning, possible blame or scapegoating	Double-loop learning including examining values, beliefs, attitudes, and behaviours, open culture about making errors and how we learn from them
Focus on technical skills	Focus on non-technical and technical skills. Invest in communication skills, team training, and human factors

We have been told in various reports (including the Francis[16] and Berwick[17] reports) and through the trial by media that followed the publication of these reports that the NHS has lost its empathy. I disagree; I know many wonderful caring people across the NHS who work tirelessly for the benefit of others. There might be the odd bad apple but these people are rare, the exception and not the rule. There are, however, some problems with the system within which we work and also some cultural issues.

Wherever I visit, across the UK, north and south, GPs, district general and larger hospitals, I hear the effects of the target-driven culture that has been imposed upon us. To enable us to be the caring empathic people that I believe us to be, we need *time*.

I hear again and again that we are understaffed (either insufficient numbers, poor skill mix, or both); this means that we are time poor which in turn means that we are fire-fighting all the time. Consequently some of the sacrifices that are commonly made are on the niceties.

I do not believe that any NHS member of staff gets out of bed in the morning with an 'I don't care' attitude. Somehow we need to free people up so that they have time to deliver the care they would like to give. I would like to offer five tips to do just this.

Tip 1: Streamline processes and decrease duplication, freeing up time

How can you streamline processes for your staff to free them up to care? Why is it that all the data collection that they have to do for different agencies and governing bodies overlaps and duplicates itself? Why can't we decide to amalgamate these so we can collect one set of data? How can you push a decision to do this back up the management chain? Which systems can we simplify so there is less time filling in forms and ticking boxes and more time at the bedside? Do the clinicians need to be the form-fillers, or can we delegate that task responsibly to others so that we can free up the clinicians to care for patients (see Example 7.1)?

Example 7.1 Orthopaedic joint-injection clinic

I will illustrate this last question with an example. In one clinic the orthopaedic consultant has an overbooked list of joint injections every week. Let us say for the sake of this example that it was agreed that it was feasible to do ten joint injections in the time allocated and there are usually at least 14 patients booked in. The consultant has a theatre list immediately after the clinic and must start on time or patients will be cancelled from that list. If the particular paperwork or electronic record in the clinic is not recorded and coded correctly, the fee for the procedure isn't paid. This is a laborious process that even in swift hands takes a minimum of seven minutes (if the computer is in a co-operative mood).

The consultant seems to face some choices:

Option 1—complete all 14 procedures and over-run by an hour with the extra four patients, but don't fill in any of the paperwork.

Option 2—complete all the paperwork but manage only nine patients in the same time of a one hour over-run. This would mean cancelling five patients

---

who would all need an explanation, an apology, and a new date, all of which would take more time.

The consultants who conduct the clinic opt for option 1. They put the patients first and say 'to hell with the paperwork!' Not surprisingly, the ops manager for this area is rather unhappy as his service, which is very productive where people are working very hard, is not receiving any income.

What other options can you consider?

Of course, there are many possible solutions to this (more consultant time, change timetables, alter commissioning processes, update IT systems so they are quicker, run a long waiting list and use it as a stick—I am *not* advocating the last one—and so on.). Here is one of mine I'd like you to consider.

Employ a band 2 administrator to fill in the paperwork: the new staff member would pay for him or herself because the organization would actually be paid for the procedures he or she is completing. This person could also help with some of the other tasks within the clinic and improve overall efficiency. This would be cheaper than paying for the consultant to do the same task and the consultant may actually finish earlier and get to the theatre list on time. Without the constant time pressure the consultant will be able to focus better on operating and may even be less likely to make a mistake. This takes us back to *making it easy for people to do the right thing*. Expecting someone to assess all of the pre-operative patients too quickly so that he or she can start the operating list and then try to operate quicker than advisable is not a recipe for safety.

Have you asked your staff what gets in the way of things being efficient?

Have you listened?

What have you all learned?

More importantly, have you acted on this information?

Tip 2: Eliminate the 'fluffy bunny' allergy and recruit for values

There is a subset within the current cultural trends that I find rather disturbing— the concept of non-technical skills (communication skills, team working, and all of the contents of the G-NO-TECS framework) being too 'fluffy'. This exists in pockets or in micro-cultures.

If I try to stay curious about where this response comes from, I find the underlying thoughts and emotions difficult to fathom. Perhaps it is a defensive or avoidance response because thinking about non-technical skills is on the 'too-hard' pile for those people with a low EQ. Perhaps it is not exciting enough as it doesn't involve a fancy bit of kit or learning a practical skill. Perhaps it is because we can't measure these skills easily and that we are told that data and measurement are everything. Some people may have a preference for logic, thinking rather than emotion, perhaps influenced by their personality styles. However, we cannot hide behind our personality preference. It is just that, a preference. Behaviour is a choice. Some behaviours will be easier for some people than others. You don't, however, get to opt out. We have traditionally employed some professional groups of people because of their purported high intelligence. We will continue to employ highly intelligent staff but I hope we will also consider their emotional intelligence (Box 7.1).

Box 7.1 Soap-box moment

*If you find yourself tempted to fall into the, 'I don't do touchy feely' category then learn! We are in health**care**. The **care** is in there for a reason.*

Empathy does not involve performing a procedure, or an admission, or a clinic attendance that helps to hit targets.

You cannot easily measure empathy and caring. You simply feel it. I do not expect to hear the phrase 'so where is the evidence when considering care or empathy'!

So where is the evidence?'

We ought to **recruit** for values too. In the future I hope we will also **promote** with values in mind. There are a number of people in senior leadership roles who are not good role models. I hope that among the values we seek we will include emotional intelligence!

Tip 3: Distributive leadership (eliminate command and control)

I want to return to the idea of shared responsibility for change. If we are going to achieve culture change then it has be something that everyone brings about because it is the very 'way we do things around here' that needs to change.

The way that we teach human factors ensures that everyone who attends a course, no matter what their grade or hierarchical position, offers a new idea for change. We help everyone who attends our course to come up with an idea and to identify what the first steps might be towards realizing it. This triggers a series of new ideas which crop up all over the organization. It also gives people permission to think about improving things for themselves. They don't have to wait for someone else to tell them to do this. No matter what their grade we want their ideas, we want to listen to them and we want to invest time in helping them make their idea become a reality. They know the challenges they face, so they can find a tailor made solution.

I had a wonderful moment the other day when the eyes of a junior staff nurse from ICU lit up at the end of one of my courses and she proudly announced that she felt *she* could change something. She had never realized that before. She grew metaphorically in front of me. It was wonderful feedback.

Tip 4: Daily debrief

I believe that the daily debrief can be part of the change process that helps us introduce a learning culture. By taking the time to ask a few pertinent questions at the end of our shifts we can make tiny changes every day. If we all make tiny improvements every day, or even every week, the net direction of travel is positive.

Daily debriefing helps us with double-loop learning. We can explore the values, attitudes, and behaviours underlying our actions. With that knowledge we can plan beneficial, long-term changes rather than just superficial quick fixes.

Tip 5: Human factors training for all

It is my firm belief that we need to invest in training everyone across the NHS in human factors. This training has the capacity to underpin the shift that we need to see towards a learning culture. It moves the emphasis in our work towards a better understanding of the components of SHEEP, including: leadership, followership, and team working, of decision making, of both situational and self-awareness, and of information transfer. We know that human factors are what underlie most of our errors, so why wouldn't we want to make improvements?

I have dedicated the last chapter of the book to sharing what we have learned over the last five years (at the time of writing) as we have delivered this training. I want to share what we have learned so that others do not have to reinvent a wheel that is already in motion.

I am not deluded enough to think that we can eliminate all the errors that human beings make but I believe we can improve on we are doing now. By implementing human factors training for everyone in healthcare, I believe we can improve safety, improve patient care, and improve how we work together and look after each other.

Key points (up to and including Chapter 7)

- Situational awareness can be considered as having three components:

  - perception (***what?***),

  - comprehension (***so what?***), and

  - predicting future state (***what next?***).

- We make sense of what we have perceived so that it becomes a working mental model.

- When working in a team it is important that the ***mental model*** is shared with, and shared by, the team members. Remember patients' relatives and carers are our team members too.

- Remember that ***commentating*** is a skill where we speak our thoughts out loud. This not only slows our thinking down and makes it more deliberate; it also helps to control our stress levels and helps others to understand what we thinking. The latter links to generating a shared mental model.

- This shared mental model builds towards a team situational assessment or problem definition.

- Barriers to perception and comprehension include:

  - high workload,

  - time pressure,

  - perceived high risk,

  - stress,

  - fatigue,

  - biases (including expectation, confirmation, and environmental), and

  - task fixation.

- When building our mental model problems can arise due to:

  - missed cues,

  - misinterpreting cues, or

  - choosing to ignore cues,

  - incorrect risk assessment,

- poor time judgement, or

- a failure to update our mental model either when new information becomes available or when conditions change.

- It can be useful to do a quick run through of **SHEEP** to help with situational awareness.

  - S—which guideline/SOP are we using? Do we have all of the information we need?

  - H—who is doing what? How is that working? Is someone time keeping?

  - E—are we in the best place for what we are facing?

  - E—do we have all the kit that we need?

  - P—how full is my bucket? Where is my focus?

- Once we have completed our situational assessment or problem definition we move on to asking '*what are we going to do about it?*'

- There are four main types of decision-making process:

  - *recognition-primed or intuitive,*

  - *rule-based,*

  - *option generation*, and

  - *creative*.

- How we decide which method suits the situation depends on time pressure, risk, and the novelty of the situation.

- The rule-based approach for emergencies exists to make life easier for us.

- When we have more time we can use an option generation model such as DECIDE.

- Making a decision is only the first step in a cycle. We should then continuously monitor that treatment or plan and review it. This is especially true in the light of new information.

- It is vital to update our mental model with new information.

- Please guard against the *assumption* that the diagnosis is definitely correct.

- We need to spend more time reviewing how we are making our decisions so that we can improve this skill.

- Conflict can be considered as an **unmet need**.

- Conflict can be classed as substantive or personal.

- Substantive conflict has a place in change or in moving things forward. It isn't always negative.

- It is worth understanding the conflict triangle: people—who is fighting and where are the clashes; process—how does the conflict manifest itself; and the underlying problem—what are they fighting about?

- When personal conflict occurs, in understanding people, it is worth unpicking why it has occurred and trying to understand it in terms of MBTI styles, preferred learning styles (Honey and Mumford), and preferred team roles (Belbin).

- When helping to resolve conflict some basic tools are useful: listening skills, perfecting your 'interested', open questioning, and an understanding of eye contact, posture, stillness, and planning the environment.

- The next important skill is mastering your 'attention'. Improvement with this skill can be helped with mindfulness.

- Other skills that are useful to develop in these settings are self-awareness, self-management, and the management of your own value and belief system.

- Other skills to acquire include summarizing, reflecting back, positive reframing, hypothesis, pre-framing, prompts, clarifying questions, and appreciative enquiry.

- A mediator may be necessary and very helpful in resolving some conflicts.

- Some of the additional tools a mediator may use include 'normalizing', 'mutualizing', past-to-future state, concatenation, and a skilful use of positive reframing.

- Hierarchy management has an important role in conflict resolution.

- The graded assertiveness tool CUSS can be useful when you need to highlight a concern but don't know quite how to tackle the subject. The acronym stands for Concern, Unsure, Safety, and Stop.

- Once conflict has been resolved, there needs to be some time invested in developing the team.

- Coaching has a role to play in both individual and team development.

- A commonly used approach in coaching is TGROW: Topic, Goal, Reality, Options, and Will/Wrap up.

- When considering team development it can be helpful to use Hawkins' approach: CLEAR (contracting, listening, exploring, action, and review).

- Hawkins suggests the team look at external fit, internal focus, how they will work together, and who else will the team work with.

- Lencione suggests there are five main causes of a dysfunctional team:

  - absence of trust,

  - fear of conflict,

  - lack of commitment,

  - avoidance of accountability, and

  - inattention to results.

- Debriefing helps us achieve double-loop learning.

- Honey and Mumford describe four preferred learning styles: activists, pragmatists, theorists, and reflectors.

- We need to cater to all learning styles.

- There are a number of debriefing models to use as a framework. I use the traffic-cone method of vent, description, analysis, generalize/apply to real situations.

- Useful techniques include 80:20, open questions, appreciative enquiry, use of silence, summarizing, reflect back, hypothesis, pre-framing, paraphrasing, and 'normalizing'.

- We should all aim for a daily debrief, even if we work on our own. 'What did I learn today?' 'How will that change what I do in the future?'

- After-action review is another simple framework.

- My slightly adapted version of the after-action review is:

  - **what did you expect to happen?**

  - **what actually happened?**

  - **what are the differences between these?**

  - **how do you think they came about? Consider SHEEP.**

  - **what have we learned?**

- Modern thoughts on leadership go beyond trait theories and heroic leadership.

- Goffee suggests successful leaders show vulnerability, are happy to be different, demonstrate tough empathy, and are great at reading a situation.

- Kotter suggests that management produces order and consistency. He describes planning, budgeting, staffing, organizing, controlling, and problem solving as management activities.

- Kotter suggests that leadership focuses on producing change. The parallel activities for leadership are described as vision building, strategy, aligning people, communicating, motivating, and inspiring.

- Ancona advocates sense making, relating, visioning, and inventing but acknowledges that these skills do not have to be found in one individual and can be the result of a team effort.

- Heifetz usefully proposes the metaphor of the balcony and the dance floor, identification of the adaptive challenges, regulating distress, maintaining disciplined attention, leaving responsibility for the adaptive challenges with the whole team, and protecting the voices from below.

- Culture can most simply be described as 'the way we do things around here'.

- We need to think of our role as having two aspects: we do our job and we improve how we do our job.

- Heifetz encourages us to think of leadership as learning and to ask '*who needs to learn what in order to develop, understand, commit to, and implement the strategy?*'

- Whilst we may all have a preferred learning style (pragmatist, activist, theorist, or reflector), we all need to be able to learn from experience.

- In the simplest terms when we work, we perform a combination of 'doing', 'thinking', 'understanding theory', and 'experimenting'.

- Learning that develops capability takes place when we engage with something uncertain and unfamiliar.

- We need to shift perspectives, question assumptions, and reappraise expectations.

- By applying existing knowledge and competencies in a novel way we can adapt to new situations.

◆ It is only when we start to acknowledge the complexity and ambiguity that we face and apply an adaptive approach that we will start to succeed in rising to the challenges of providing high-quality healthcare.

References

1. Senge PM. *The Fifth Discipline: The Art and Practice of the learning Organization*, 1990.
2. Drucker PF, Dyson E, Handy C, et al. Looking Ahead: Implications of the Present. *Harvard Business Review* 1997; 75 (5): 18–32.
3. Cook D. Culture and Organizational Learning. *Journal of Management Inquiry* 1993; 2: 373–90.
4. Honey P. *The Learning Styles Questionnaire: 80-item version*. Maidenhead: Peter Honey Publications, 2006.
5. Argyris C, Schon DA. *Theory in Practice: Increasing Professional Effectiveness*. San Francisco, CA: Jossey-Bass, 1974.
6. Kolb DA. *Experiential Learning: Experience as the Source of Learning and Development*. Englewood Cliffs, NJ: Prentice Hall, 1984.
7. Gibbs G. *Learning by Doing: A Guide to Teaching and Learning Methods*. Oxford: Oxford Centre for Staff and Learning Development, Oxford Brookes University, 1988.
8. Grant J and Marsden P. *Training Senior House Officers by Service-based Training*. Joint Conference for Education in Medicine. London, 1992. *British Medical Journal* 1989; 299: 1263–68.
9. Seaman DF, Fellenz RA. *Effective Strategies for Teaching Adults*. Columbus, OH: Merrill Publishing Co., 1989.
10. Luft J. *Group processes: an introduction to group dynamics*, 3rd edn. Mountain View, CA: Mayfield, 1984.
11. Bloom BS. *Taxonomy of Educational Objectives: The Classification of Educational Goals. Handbook 1: Cognitive Domain*. London: Longmans, Green & Co., 1956.
12. Engelhart MD, Bloom BS. *Cognitive Domain*. New York, NY: McKay, 1956.
13. Krathwohl DR, Bloom BS, Masia BB. *Taxonomy of Educational Objectives: The Classification of Educational Goals: Handbook 2: Affective Domain*. London: Longmans, Green & Co., 1956.
14. Krathwohl DR. *Taxonomy of Educational Objective.: The Classification of Educational Goals*. London: Longmans Green, 1964.
15. Kirkpatrick DL. *Evaluating Training Programs: The Four Levels*: San Francisco, CA: Berrett-Koehler Publishers, 1994.
16. Francis R. 2013 Final Report of the Mid Staffordshire NHS Foundation Trust Public Inquiry. Available at: <http://www.midstaffspublicinquiry.com/report>.
17. Berwick D. A Promise to Learn—A Commitment to Act. Improving the Safety of Patients in England: National Advisory Group on the Safety of Patients in England, 2013. Available at: <https://www.gov.uk/government/uploads/system/.../Berwick_Report.pdf>.

8

Teaching human factors in healthcare

Tell me and I will forget.
Show me and I may remember.
But involve me and I will understand.

Japanese proverb

Sharing our experience

At the time of writing in early 2014, we have been running stand-alone human factors courses on two levels for a range of professionals for over five years. The advanced level is run monthly; the basic level is now running weekly.

Of course, there are many ways to teach this topic and what I share with you here are only *my* thoughts. I have already made it clear that I think it is time for us to have taken on board the learning from the airline industry but to have moved beyond it. I believe that the human factors we teach, should be 'aeroplane free' and instead should be packed full of healthcare examples. It is on these principles that I have run my courses.

Whilst we include human-factors training in every simulation debrief that we run, I want to move into the realms of pure, stand-alone, human-factors training. I will not delve into the importance of winning over the executive board and the governors and writing business cases here but it is important to know that these were the first steps in my experience. If you are going to be successful launching human factors training across your own organization it essential to get yourself some high-level enthusiasts (at least an executive sponsor) within the organization to support your efforts. With the Human Factors Concordat[1] that was issued in November 2013, I hope that it will be considerably easier to foster executive 'buy in' to the importance of the training.

In addition to high-level backing there are other things to consider which will, I hope, greatly assist your progress.

Debbie's top tips
Who will you need?

1. Great administrative support is a vital component to education and it is top of my list for a reason. Efficient, effective administration happens quietly behind the scenes. Without it, it is not possible to run effective courses. You need to budget for a good administrator's time.

2. Faculty—I am very fussy when selecting staff for facilitating human factors in particular, because I think they should act as role models for the behaviours we are advocating (e.g. approachable leaders, good listening, positive outlook, self-awareness, ability to share how they learned from their own mistakes, etc.). We need facilitation for these courses, not top-down instruction. I want my faculty to be curious, to look for the right questions to ask, and question the answers. In my opinion, human-factors training is not suitable for novice facilitators. Would-be facilitators ought to 'cut their educational teeth' on something easier before they move to cultural and behavioural change.

For whom?
Multi-professional courses (please!)

A large number of healthcare related errors occur when there is a break down in information flow across specialties and professions. By mixing people from different professional groups when we train, we can bring down some of the 'us and them' inter-professional boundaries and encourage the removal of silo working. All of our courses are attended by roughly one-third medical, a slightly more than one-third nursing, midwifery, and allied health professionals, and one-third non-clinical individuals.

Everyone in healthcare, no matter what their role, should be trained in human factors at the basic level. We train medics from registrar level, nursing and allied health professionals at band 7 and higher (or band 6 or lead a team), and non-clinical at band 6 and above on our advanced course.

Do they jump or are they pushed?

As I suspect any educator will confirm, it is far easier to teach those who have come willingly rather than those who are 'sent'. When we started, we had a flurry of enthusiasts. We worked hard to engage people, to get them excited, and we developed a sense of anticipation in those who heard about the course from others. A large proportion of the early attendees were in educational roles themselves. Once we were up and running, the course became self-sustaining.

Participants from the two-day course would sing its praises to their peers and encourage their teams to attend the half-day course. Word of mouth is a powerful persuader.

People react to change differently: some embrace it, others are not so sure, and some sub-specialties are more prepared for it than others. We were soon running a waiting list for a place on the course. In a number of specialties we came across the notion that the topic was 'soft skills' and therefore not particularly important. Knowledge and technical skills were mistakenly considered the only important aspect of training amongst some sub-groups. For me, of course, the technical and non-technical skills are inextricably linked. You can have all of the knowledge and skills that you like, but if you can't draw on them at the right time, share your mental model of the treatment plan with your team, and know how to reduce your chance of making errors, your patient will not be receiving the best possible care.

Where?

Venue

Give some thought to where you train people. If possible, try to choose somewhere that will allow people to think differently from their normal day-to-day routine. We are trying to alter perception with this training, not simply trying to teach facts and figures. Behavioural change is a different level of training than knowledge and skills training, and the setting plays an important part in ensuring the training is effective. I realize that within the limited budgets of the NHS we cannot recreate the 'thinking spaces' some major corporations have at their disposal, but try to make the location somewhere stimulating and away from the clinical environment if you can.

How long and how often?

We run a half-day basic course and an advanced two-day course. The 'train the trainer' course lasts for five days, and it assumes that you have prior teaching experience.

How often is harder to judge and I can't yet offer a definitive answer, although I am happy to report that people do ask when they can come back. It is worth bearing in mind that the aviation industry mandates annual human factors updates.

We send a monthly update with a short patient story, or a scenario with a tongue-in-cheek mini-quiz, or just a reminder to all those who have attended a course.

How?

Interactive

I ban the use of PowerPoint™ on my courses. This forces educators to be more inventive. I want the sessions to be not only engaging but involving and I am a firm believer in experiential learning; I don't want simply to talk about information transfer, I want people to experience what I am discussing. They have to have the opportunity to make mistakes but then to understand why. I want them to experience interruptions when they are performing a task and realize how frustrating this can be and how it interferes with their ability to stay focused on their primary objective. We can then link this to the next time they are tempted to interrupt the nurse doing the drug round.

I want attendees to be performing a task in isolation without understanding the point of the whole exercise so that in future, they will spend more time making sure their own team members are more aware of how their role is important and how it fits into the whole.

Small groups

For me this is vital. When we started we religiously had a maximum of 12 delegates. As time has passed and we became more confident with the course material and how we run the course, we have allowed numbers to rise to around 16. I am adamant though that human factors is not the sort of thing that can be covered in a didactic way. It does not lend itself to either lectures nor to e-learning. Each person needs time to talk, to share their experiences, and to practise techniques. They need time to listen to other people's experiences, too. This is how we bring down any inter-professional barriers. Hearing about someone else's experiences and sensing how they felt about them is not the same as watching it on a screen. You can interact with them and ask questions. The facilitator can extract lessons to be learned while checking that everyone feels secure and safe, and everyone understands what is being learned.

It is also a very different experience doing something rather than having someone tell you the principles of how to do it.[2]

Multiple formats

Each part of the course or mini-session only lasts a maximum of 40–50 minutes. This is then followed by a micro-break, and then by a change of teaching format.

Knowing what we do about the limited attention span of the human mind is important; I am a strong advocate of changing formats to maintain people's interest. We are also aware that we all learn differently. Think back to the camera metaphor used to illustrate Honey and Mumford[3] (Chapter 5) or to Kolb[4] and the other educational theories (Chapter 7).

You can change many aspects of the training session: a change of media, room layout, group size (working as a whole group or in pairs, then coming back together again), change of tempo, change of emotional content (serious and hard-hitting sessions followed by something fun and lighter), problem solving and drawing on one's own experience to being given information which one must assimilate and then give back to the rest of the group, physically moving about rather than just remaining seated. I think this variety keeps people engaged.

Strong ice-breaking techniques and a safe environment

I am convinced that when we work in multi-professional groups with people who do not know each other and are not used to being trained together, ice-breaking at the beginning is vital. If we are to learn together to the extent that we are altering perceptions, we need to build a feeling of trust in the room and a 'safe' learning environment. This does not happen by accident. It takes a good deal of focus and skilled facilitation.

What do I mean by ice breaking? I mean that everyone has spoken and revealed a little bit of something personal about themselves. There has been time for a few laughs and a bit of empathy. I need to feel that any hierarchies in the room have been levelled off, including any perceived ones about me. I never introduce myself by my title; I am simply Debbie or Debs (Professor Rosenorn-Lanng sounds rather less approachable). I reveal my love of coffee and chocolate. I share something about having six children. On the advanced course (when we have more time), I also tell a story of my first weekend on call which I will share with you now.

It was my first house job. My first rota on call fell on a weekend. In those days (yes, I promised I would not become one of those older consultants who reminisced about 'in my day' but ...) we worked long weekends, from Friday morning to Monday night. On the Friday night I finally finished what I was doing and managed to get to bed. No one had told me about going to bed in 'blues', so I happily put on my silk pyjamas and climbed in. Not long after, there was a crash call to A&E. I ended up in A&E in my silk pyjamas and was regularly reminded of this for the next six months!

Storytelling

I am a strong advocate of telling stories drawn from real life. I think they are very powerful, particularly if they are local and relevant. They, of course, need to be handled sensitively and with care because they can trigger profound emotional responses.

The case of Elaine Bromiley is currently available online, and further information about her case is available on the CHFG (clinical human-factors group) website.[7]

There are companies that provide stories on DVD (for example, see <http://www.patientstories.org.uk>[8]).

Local stories are also very powerful and promote organizational learning but they need to be handled sensitively and they need to be anonymous. The focus needs to be on the learning and not on blaming. A useful approach is to invest in filming a role play of a local scenario. Handle it with care by changing the names and some of the details but be true to the learning.

Participants' own examples

Encouraging participants to share their own experience also needs to be facilitated carefully. There need to be some ground rules introduced covering not using people's real names and respecting confidentiality on the course. We always ask people to take away the learning and to share it as widely as possible but to leave the specifics of any local case in the room. This can be a bit of a balancing act but I believe that local examples are very relevant and powerful tools to use.

Sharing real-life examples can give someone the opportunity to vent, to be debriefed and supported, and to learn from the event him or herself. Lessons can then be captured by everyone in the room and shared. I find that this often triggers recall of parallel stories and experiences from other participants, and this helps to unite people from different professional groups when they can see that they face the same challenges as others.

Positivity

I expend a lot of energy on my courses generating a feeling of 'can do' and a 'glass-half-full' approach. We spend time talking about how important it is to 'ban the Mood Hoover'. We discuss raising morale and how this can improve both mortality and morbidity. The conversations include the effects of smiling, simple acts of kindness, and the use of language. It also involves challenging any negativity that the group puts forward.

Challenge and curiosity

I challenge any sweeping generalizations and any statements that serve to reinforce the silo working of professional groups. I challenge negativity, stereotypes, assumptions, and defensive responses.

The reason that human-factors training is not the realm of the novice facilitator is the emotive nature of some of the topics. If we are really going to explore such intensely personal topics such as conflict, whose buttons we push, and examples of poor behaviour and mistakes that we have made, this may elicit an emotional response from some individuals. It is our role to be aware of these reactions, to challenge preconceptions, to try to raise awareness about assumptions, to encourage reflection on difficult situations, and to watch both individuals within the group and the group behaviour itself as well as to maintaining our own balcony view of how emotions are playing out in the room. I find that remaining curious about peoples' reactions rather than assuming I know why they answered in a certain way is essential.

I actively encourage the group to remain curious when they interact with their team, other staff, or patients. Sneak up onto the dance floor[5] during all of your encounters and ask yourself what is going on in the interaction you are observing? If you spot a certain response in someone else, don't assume that you know what it means; ask them (see Example 8.1).

The flipside of this particular coin is of course that people may well observe a reaction in you too and may be placing a value judgement on your behaviour (see Example 8.2).

I try to encourage participants to think if they find themselves getting angry or annoyed, 'which of my needs are not being met and how could I express that need?' Be curious about yourself. Ask, 'what is going on for me right now?'

Example 8.1 Observations coupled with questions

1. 'My comment seemed to evoke a response in you. What are your thoughts/feelings/ideas?'

   Comment: Does someone look angry or upset? Don't assume this to be the case. It may be that for them, this is simply how they express their passion for a topic.

2. 'I am conscious we haven't heard from everyone. Is there anything we have missed?'

   Comment: One person looking withdrawn can be another person's way of being reflective or thoughtful. Avoid the assumption.

Example 8.2 Help others not to make assumptions by being open-minded

1. I have an 'E' preference on my MBTI (Myers–Briggs type indicator). This contributes to my natural tendency to talk myself through something and commentate on my actions. I like to bounce ideas around with others. I tend to think out loud. I am aware that I do it. If I think I am working with a group with a strong 'I' MBTI preference, I will work hard to stay quiet. I will focus on listening with invisible tape over my mouth.

   This 'staying quiet, listening me' is a persona that I have had to develop for my coaching and debriefing, when ideally I only allow myself to be talking 20 per cent of the time, or less.

   In my early days of coaching, people who knew me well prior to the coaching would comment on 'how quiet I had been. Was I alright?'

   I have learned to brief people before I start coaching that I am quite different when coaching than the lively person that I might be at other times.

2. I talk louder and become quite animated when I am excited about something. This can be misconstrued. I now try to warn people about this (or, on a good day, even manage to rein it in when I can remain mindful).

Empathy and feelings are to be encouraged

The emphasis should be on care and compassion, not on targets. We need to make it easy for people to do the right thing and this includes living up to the values that I believe are universally held across the NHS: patient care first. We need to talk about this issue, prioritize it, look at who offers the best role models for it, and give it the attention it deserves. We need to challenge the things that are getting in the way of our values and our natural tendency to care. By spending time talking about this in the training sessions we are putting patient care firmly back on the radar. I am not advocating trying to teach empathy; I am talking about raising awareness of what might be getting in the way.

Openness, candour, and a learning culture

If we are advocating an open or learning culture within the human factors fraternity then it is vital that we look at role models for this within the training programme. It is important to watch the cultural barometer during told stories or scenarios and keep the issue of apportioning blame at bay, replacing it with understanding and gathering the necessary lessons from each example. This may involve the facilitator demonstrating vulnerability and admitting when he or she has made mistakes.

We have set the scene for our training programme: the importance of having small groups in an interactive, safe learning environment, all with a positive attitude, honest, and caring. It is time to move to the specifics.

I don't set any pre-course reading. The reason is that invariably within a group, some people will have completed the reading and some will not. This results in an uneven playing field before the course has even begun. The options are then to go over the pre-course material and risk boring the more studious attendees, or to assume that you can start with the pre-course material under everyone's belt and lose those who haven't done the reading. My preference is that we will deliver everything required on the course and then follow up with more detail and an ongoing drip feed of information, as the course is only the beginning. The real learning comes when attendees apply new knowledge and behaviours in real working life.

What follows won't be enough for you to start running your own course but it might give you a flavour of what we think is important. Our courses have been modified many, many times, and I am keen to share some of what we have learned so that others don't have to start from scratch.

After running through our course content, I will include some key factors that have been identified by various groups that I work with and from our course that I think should be covered in all human factors training.

Basic course

Introduction

Having looked at ice-breaking techniques and run a background check of what everyone already knows (or thinks they don't know) about human factors, we establish what each attendee would like to get out of the session. We link this to the learning objectives that we have planned.

This is standard educational practice, not rocket science. It sounds easy but remember this is the vital part where you are setting up the safe learning environment so that everyone feels able to contribute and to share errors in a non-judgemental way. Give this plenty of time.

New idea: stage 1

We introduce the importance of everyone generating an idea to change something in their own workplace. We ask people to think about something that annoys them about where they work. 'Is there something at work that makes you think there is a better way to do that?' We emphasize that this could be a very small personal thing or something much larger. We help them to identify what the first step towards this change might be. The emphasis is on patient benefit but this does not mean that our course attendees have to be directly interacting with patients. Everyone is on the course for the same reason, to benefit patients.

Throughout the course when people mention problems and issues in their own workplace we capture these on a flipchart for later discussion.

Stickies on a stickman

The first exercise that we run allows people to explore what factors may contribute to an error during their working day. The exercise continues with each participant giving examples of what makes their day run really smoothly, or the flipside—if these things are not in place, how the result can be a very negative day. This helps break the ice a little further. We spend a few minutes with each person using a coaching technique to draw out topics including what the difference is between communication and information flow, interruptions and how to manage them, what makes a team work well together, the effects of fatigue and stress. Common themes emerge no matter which professions and specialties are represented in the group. We highlight how difficult it is to remember all of the topics when they are presented at random.

At this point we introduce the concept of the SHEEP sheet and tell participants that after a break we will help to pull all of these random factors together in a memorable way. Having put up a picture of a SHEEP somewhere along their route into the training room, we ask how many have seen it at this point. This is our first link to situation awareness.

Micro-break.

The SHEEP sheet

We briefly introduce the sections of the SHEEP model sharing a few examples from each. We ask them to map their earlier examples to sections of SHEEP.

We ask our participants to think back to the last error made that they can remember. We ask them to tick any boxes on the SHEEP sheet that were relevant on that occasion. When they have finished we ask them to count the ticks. The current range is 5–77, with a mean of 25.

We use this illustration for two reasons. In the first instance we discuss James Reason's Swiss-cheese concept and how there are multiple factors involved in errors. We point out the flaw of root-cause analysis if it seeks to find only a single-point solution. We spend some time discussing work-arounds, streamlining processes, and safety. We also highlight the need to move away from waiting for the error to happen and *then* looking for lessons to be learned, and the importance of moving towards proactive looking for where an error might occur and trying to prevent it *before* it happens. This increases error awareness and SHEEP awareness. We introduce the concept of briefing and how the team might use this time to think about where an error might crop up. On a given day, if the team starts to see the ticks building up it is time to put in extra checks and seek to prevent the error, don't just wait for it!

Micro-break.

Case study: Elaine Bromiley or 'just a routine operation'—a film

I often introduce this film (see Level One, Introduction, p. x) from dual personal standpoints of having been an anaesthetist but also having had sinus surgery. I highlight a couple of technical issues for the non-clinicians in the room but point out that I want people to watch non-technical skills and so encourage them to observe the behaviours and interactions.

I debrief on the film using an open-questioning technique. I allow participants to choose what they wish to discuss and then draw out lessons to be learned from their observations. If they have missed things that I consider to be important this is again highlighted through questions. In general, the lessons derived from this are extensive. The topics that I like to have covered are included here.

Systems

◆ Error chains

◆ Guidelines and SOPs (standard operating procedures)

   ○ Why we might fail to use these

   ○ How might we help others to use them when required

   ○ Storage and access to cognitive aids, and their use

◆ Culture

Human interaction

◆ Hierarchy

   ○ Flat hierarchy and leadership

   ○ Steep hierarchy, assertion and approachability

   ○ Encouraging everyone in team to generate options and share ideas

   ○ CUSS

- Commentating and shared mental model
- Naming the emergency/making the diagnosis and decision making
- Role allocation
  - Doing versus leading, seeing the big picture
  - Time keeping
  - Feedback about observations and vital signs
  - Use of cognitive aids
- Information transfer
  - Read back
  - Making sure you are heard
- Group behaviour and complacency (think of smelling smoke in a group)

Environment

- Expectation bias regarding where you are (day case, private sector versus acute emergency-department setting)
- Situational awareness and the influence of where you are located

Equipment

- Familiarity with equipment and when to use it (not just how to use it)

Personal

- Expectation bias in a routine setting, complacency versus always being prepared and expecting the unexpected

Another micro-break is followed by something more active.

The drawing task

In much the same way as I asked you to draw a house by component parts in Level One, we use a drawing task to illustrate the potential flaws to be found in information transfer and offer tips to ensure these traps are avoided.

We divide the group into pairs of people who do not know each other and who have completely different backgrounds. The choice of partner is left to those in the room and we leave them to sort it out for as long as it takes. What they do not realize is they are selecting their buddy. We will come to the role of the buddy later.

We ask each pair to sit back to back, therefore robbing them of the possibility of non-verbal communication. To one person in the pair we give a picture. On the left-hand side of that picture is a list of words they are not allowed to use when describing the picture. The second person is given drawing materials. The first simply has to describe the picture and second has to draw it. At the end of the task we ask the group to re-form but for each pair to sit next to each other.

As we debrief the task, we ask each pair to do the equivalent of the primary school 'show and tell', or you can think of it as a 'before and after'.

The topics that we pull out from the session include the following:

◆ Non-verbal versus verbal communication

◆ Face to face versus phone versus email, texting, and written communication

◆ Big picture versus detail, and links to MBTI

◆ Funnelling

◆ Information transfer

◆ Read back

◆ Clarification

◆ Shared mental model

◆ Assumption

◆ Personal differences in information transfer

The assumptions discovered at this stage are fascinating. Invariably, within the group some will have been made. Usually, a number of those drawing will assume that they cannot speak to their partner and so information will have flowed in one direction without read back or clarification. Others will be surprised to see that the other person has drawn something completely different from what they expected to see. All in all, this particular task is extremely revealing for all involved.

Encourage reflection on lessons learned thus far.

Micro-break.

Structured information tool

Our preference is to use SBAR (situation, background, assessment, recommendation/request), although RSVP (reason, story, vital signs, plan) or another tool would work just as well (I have to say that as a community I do think we should standardize the use of tools like these nationally). After a brief introduction to the tool, we then present a very jumbled paragraph of written information filled with red herrings and irrelevant facts. We have devised both a clinical and a non-clinical version of this. There is a crisis situation in each scenario offered, with multiple logistical challenges. The pair must perform an analysis sorting out the 'wood from the trees', entering this information into the correct part of the SBAR tool.

By using the tool to tackle a logistical problem, it avoids the need for everyone to have clinical knowledge. It highlights the strength of a tool which people traditionally think of as being used solely to hand over a single patient.

The lessons that we try to highlight are as follows:

◆ Benefits and adaptability of a structured tool

◆ The tool can be used to extract information as well as deliver it

◆ The importance of prioritization and filtering information

◆ Emphasis on funnelling

◆ Phone calls being an at-risk time of information transfer

◆ Multi-professional information transfer hazards

◆ Handover risks

◆ The problems generated by Chinese whispers

Micro-break.

Activity

We use a couple of interactive activities at this point to appeal to different learning styles but also to change tempo and format in order to maintain attention.

The first activity emphasizes the following lesson:

◆ Don't set your team unrealistic targets. If you do, you risk the occurrence of:

  ○ blame

  ○ chaos and lack of leadership or direction

  ○ frustration

  ○ disengagement

  ○ in-fighting

  ○ opt out

We contrast this with a positive activity immediately afterwards aimed at experiencing:

◆ trust

◆ a safe environment for everyone to put forward their ideas

- option generation
- continuous improvement
- resilience
- motivation, buy in, and engagement
- shared goals and shared understanding
- role allocation
- listening
- what it is like to work in a good team
- leadership and 'followership'
- willingness to experiment and try new things even if they seem unlikely to work
- co-operation

Introducing the G-NO-TECS tool

On the basic level course we cover the G-NO-TECS tool superficially. It is linked to the last activity that invariably generates a sense of fun. The aspects that we highlight are read back, active identification, use of pronouns, and cross checking.

Creating change and sustainability

Generating new ideas

We explain that everyone who attends the course goes away having promised to change something. We tell participants how many people have already been through one of our courses, which encourages them to feel part of a 'change' community. The idea is that if everyone takes one tiny step forward, the overall impact is huge. We explain the buddy system at this point. Once we have generated some excitement in the room, we encourage people to come to the front and share their particular idea about change with the group. This requires positive facilitation. Some people need help to find an idea, others have so many ideas they need help to select one, but I have yet to find someone who cannot think of something. The idea ought to be cost-neutral unless finding funding is part of the idea.

Participants state their idea.

We ask each participant to fill in an ideas sheet. The sheet also has the name and contact details of their buddy. We keep this sheet. Six weeks after the course we send a photocopy of the sheet to the relevant participant. We try to get people to think of this as a trigger. We ask the buddies to meet up, in person if possible, but at the very least to pick up the phone and talk to each other. 'I received that letter from Debbie and Sue today. Have you started yet? No, me neither. We did say we would. How shall we start?'

A year later we contact everyone again to gather their successes.

We also offer both the support of a health quality-improvement team and ourselves if people get stuck. We offer some education material about PDSA (plan, do, study, act) cycles and achieving change.

Questions

Prior to closure we establish whether there are any questions that have been left unanswered.

'What question is at the forefront of your mind?'

Closure

We ask what people will take away.

We summarize key learning points that we hope they will leave with, linking these to the learning objectives. We emphasize the team nature of the human-factors community that they have now joined and we explain how we will stay in touch with them every month.

We ask for both verbal and written feedback on how we could improve the course.

Our 'happy sheet' also encourages people to think about what changes they will make in their work and what else they might need to help maintain the impetus for change. We also use a 'before and after' Likert scale to demonstrate whether there is an improvement in confidence on a list of human factors knowledge, skills, and ideas.

After the course

Reading material

We opt to do this electronically. We send out some reading material around human factors in general. We highlight the clinical human-factors group (CHFG). We now send out the Human Factors Concordat.

Drip feed

We contact all of our past participants every month with a small vignette or a bit of revision. We tell a story or set a mini quiz and try to keep the idea of human factors alive and relevant. We usually get a good number of responses from these each time.

The two-day advanced course

This course is aimed at those who are in a more managerial or leadership role. Broadly speaking, this course is aimed at medical staff (registrars and higher levels), nursing, midwifery, and allied-health professionals (at band 7 and above, unless they are a band 6 with a leadership role), and non-clinical staff (at band 6 and above).

Ice breaking

This is carried out as per the short course, but participants also choose a quote and an embarrassing moment to share. The embarrassing moment helps break the ice, and helps people get to know each other and trust one another. It encourages people to show vulnerability.

Film clip

We sometimes use a film clip of an error where a member of staff covers up for another staff member.

The lessons that we hope to pull from this include:

◆ open culture

◆ error management

◆ leadership in an emergency setting

◆ role allocation

◆ hierarchy and culture and the importance of asking for help

◆ body language and non-verbal communication

◆ situational awareness and being focused on the task at hand

◆ cover up and the implications this may have

Stickies on a stickman and SHEEP

These are both done in the same manner as on the basic course but in a bit more depth. I think it is important that if we are teaching the team on the basic course and the leader on the advanced course that there are large overlaps so that they leave us with a shared mental model of human factors and a shared language of the new terms we will use. The difference is that we have more time with the more senior ones, so we can explore topics in more depth. This increase in depth is a partially achieved by the facilitator being more probing (with open questioning), and in part due to the increased experience in the room.

SHEEP activity

We use a scenario-based task where small groups use the SHEEP sheet together.

Drawing task

This is conducted as per the basic course.

However, in the advanced course we now have more time to explore non-verbal communication. We do this in a game of charades.

Charades

We generate enthusiasm in even the most retiring soul and no-one is allowed to opt out, Christmas and sherry analogies abound. Both simple and more complex charades are included, and we use a second facilitator willing to kick things off.

We include a mixture of emotions and attitudes that we want our participants to be able to portray and perceive. We caution against making assumptions and snap judgements. We highlight the fact that we are quickly absorbing information about our patients or other members of staff, and we raise awareness about how rapidly they will be judging us.

We spend time getting everyone trying to perfect paying attention and being interested, or at very least appearing to be, when both patients and staff are talking to them.

We talk about the ease of invading someone else's personal space, and encourage participants to reflect on how a ward round is performed.

Micro-break.

Structured handover using SBAR

We sometimes use a different example from the one used on the basic course, but the principles remain the same. We want participants to be able to filter and prioritize information. We want to them to be able to process this information and categorize it. We want them to be able to apply it to the SBAR model and to have used the model in a way that is not just applicable to a single patient but for an entire situation. We link this to the funnelling principle: start with the big picture to try and establish some sort of shared mental model.

The learning objectives are the same as for the basic course.

Lunch.

Lively film clip (after lunch, in the graveyard slot)

We introduce the G-NO-TECS tool at this point. Having allowed the group to familiarize themselves briefly with the tool, we split the group in half.

Each half is given a character to observe during the film. The point is made that this part of the course is not about the technical aspects of what they observe but instead is focused on the non-technical skills contained within the G-NO-TECS tool.

The two groups then spend time comparing their character to the various components described in the tool.

We then bring those characters to life. I act the part of each character, and the relevant part of the group gives me feedback on my performance.

In addition to familiarity with and experience using the G-NO-TECS tool, the learning outcomes that we hope to highlight include:

◆ emotional intelligence and self-awareness

◆ use of clean language and body language

◆ introducing the concept of mediation

◆ using of 360-degree feedback

◆ coping with anger when it is directed at you and what to do when you feel angry

◆ a start to the topic of conflict resolution

Emotional intelligence (EQ)

We encourage participants to complete an EQ questionnaire and to reflect on their own self-awareness.

How easy would they find asking for help? How might their senior grade be a barrier to asking for help? What might they need to overcome?

No micro-break—we move quietly into the next section without any warning as I begin to speak a bit abruptly to Sue, my co-facilitator. We wait to see if the group will stop me or challenge me, but usually it dawns on them that we are hatching something together.

SBIC and challenging poor behaviour

This is achieved in the same way as on the basic course. We encourage the group to share examples of poor behaviour that they have witnessed. We teach them how to challenge this behaviour using the tried and tested tool, SBIC. We encourage people to practise using the tool for praise. Once participants have mastered the use of the tool, we praise them and suggest that the next group they try this out on are their peers. Only after lots of practice do we suggest that they move on to giving feedback to persistent offenders.

Activities

Again, these are run exactly the same as for the basic course.

Peer-led learning

From this point onwards, the advanced course becomes rather different. We introduce the concept of peer-led learning. During the lunch break, we decide how many subgroups we shall split the group into and who should work well together.

Each group is given a topic and a handout on that topic. They are then told to read the information and see which parts of it appeal to them. The idea is that their learning needs are representative of the learning needs of the group as a whole. Therefore if something appeals to them, it will probably appeal to the group also. They will share this information with the group on day 2. Each mini-group acts as a filter and processing system which will prioritize the information for the whole group.

Whilst we have given them the basics on the topic, they are free to conduct further research on topic. They are offered access to the Internet.

There are a few provisos about how the information must be delivered to the rest of the group. There is an emphasis on interactive sharing and making this part fun. PowerPoint™ is banned. Film clips are allowed. There is a time limit for the information delivery.

The subgroups start working on their topics. I float between the groups and help to plant ideas and use a few coaching techniques to encourage their ideas to blossom. Although it has not usually dawned on the participants just yet, they are practising a number of the skills we have discussed at a theoretical level. They are forming a new team. The team may need to identify its strengths and allocate roles accordingly. They need to take in information, process it, and filter and prioritize it. They need to then package that information in a way that will appeal to others and to help others to absorb it. There may be different thoughts on what the priorities should be or how the information should be shared. There may need to be time spent listening, negotiating, and compromising with others in order to achieve this. Some members of the group may be very comfortable delivering a session while others may hate it. They may need to be supportive of some members, and yet controlling with some of those who might be rather more dominant. None of this may become apparent until we get each subgroup to reflect on what has occurred during the debrief, which will happen after their session.

The session, the debrief, and the debrief of the debrief

Part of the way through day 2, I hand over the reins to the participants to run their own sessions. We conduct a rotational system. An example session is shown

Table 8.1 An example session plan

Session	Debrief	Debrief of the debrief
1	2	3 and 4
2	3	4 and 1
3	4	1 and 2
4	1	2 and 3

in Table 8.1 for four subgroups. Each subgroup chooses which slot they would like. I leave them to negotiate the order between themselves.

Following the table, group 1 runs the first interactive, fun session. Group 2 runs the first debrief session. Groups 3 and 4 run a debrief of the debrief.

The lessons to be taken from this approach occur at multiple levels simultaneously.

1. There is learning from working together in a newly formed team.

2. There is learning from the new topic.

3. There is learning associated with how to observe behaviour, how to *really* listen, and to how to break processes down using a mental framework before you debrief.

4. There is then learning how to actually do the debriefing.

I find that people have often been conditioned, Pavlov style, to deliver feedback in a judgemental way: strengths and weaknesses, good and bad, what went well, and what could be improved. It can be quite hard to move participants away from how they initially see their role as *judge* and to replace that with one of *thinking partner*.

It can take several rounds of practice to alter and replace this ingrained behaviour. Some groups grasp it more quickly than others.

Desired learning outcomes/experiences

From the team-working aspect

◆ Forming together as a new team

◆ Allowing for differences in personality, learning styles, value systems, experiences, etc., and differences in working together

◆ Role allocation

- Information gathering, filtering, sharing, and processing
- Negotiating a plan for the session
- Session delivery itself
- Working under time pressure and coping with feeling underprepared

From the session topics

We hope these will leave us with an understanding of:

- decision making,
- situational awareness,
- conflict resolution,
- 'followership', and
- leadership from the perspective of emotional intelligence.

From watching the session with a view to debriefing, or watching another team debrief

We hope attendees will work on:

- active listening (listening is not the same as waiting to speak),
- observational skills,
- learning to be aware of different needs within a group, and
- learning to spot the unspoken problem, and how to diffuse something tricky.

By learning how to debrief

Attendees will learn how to:

- establish a thinking partnership which generates a learning conversation,
- use the *vent, description, analysis, generalization model*,
- keep to the 80:20 rule when appropriate,
- work on their ratios of open to close questions,
- use layering,
- praise in a genuine and non-condescending manner,
- use hypothesis,
- use summary, paraphrasing, and reading back,
- use silence,

◆ develop a safe environment in which to explore and learn,

◆ explore the seating arrangements and understand how this might influence the feelings in the room,

◆ have a heightened awareness of the need for using clean (i.e. unambiguous) language,

◆ avoid double questions,

◆ avoid judgmental questions, and

◆ avoid closed questions, except where required for clarification.

Activity

We have designed a complex activity that runs at the beginning of day 2, building on the learning from day 1.

Attendees should both experience and learn from:

◆ problem solving,

◆ coping with ambiguity,

◆ information gathering,

◆ information transfer from one set of people to another,

◆ extracting information,

◆ coping with interference and distraction,

◆ coping with complexity and a changing workload,

◆ coping with an emergency but able to maintain routine tasks simultaneously,

◆ understanding how one's role/task fits into the whole team/task,

◆ understanding how one's team can affect other areas of an organization,

◆ read back,

◆ cross checking, and

◆ active identification.

Micro-break

I introduce the more serious aspect of the course now, in contrast to the activity that attendees have just completed. I emphasize that whilst the following event did not happen in our hospital, it occurred somewhere rather close by.

Case study: film (as per basic course but considered in greater depth)

I often introduce this film from my personal standpoint of having been an anaesthetist, but I have also been a patient who has had sinus surgery so I can offer a dual perspective.

I highlight a couple of technical issues for the non-clinicians in the room (i.e. we are taught a set sequence of actions if we 'lose' the airway; after four minutes we should cut the neck and deliver oxygen through the front of the neck. I ask attendees to watch the clock and register the time passing in the film. I also mention the concept of normal oxygen saturations and the fact that we like these to be over 94 per cent). However, I also emphasize that I want people to watch non-technical skills and encourage them to observe behaviours and inter-actions. On the advanced course, they will already be familiar with the G-NO-TECS framework. We ask people to read this again before watching the clip.

I debrief the attendees on the film using open questioning. I allow the partici-pants to choose what they wish to discuss and then extract learning from their observations. If they have missed things that I consider to be important then I highlight this using questioning. The learning from this story is extensive. The topics that I like to cover are included here.

Systems

- Error chains
- Guidelines and SOPs
  - Why we might fail to use one
  - How might we help others when they should be using one
  - Storage and access to cognitive aids and their use
- Culture
  - What is the culture like in their department
  - What might they need to do to change it

Human interaction

- Hierarchy
  - Flat hierarchy and leadership
  - Steep hierarchy and assertion and approachability
  - 15 degrees

- ○ Encouraging everyone in team to generate options and share their ideas
- ○ CUSS
- ◆ Commentating and shared mental model
- ◆ Naming the emergency/making the diagnosis, and decision making
- ◆ Role allocation
  - ○ Doing versus leading, keeping the big picture in mind
  - ○ Time keeping
  - ○ Feedback about observations and vital signs
  - ○ Use of cognitive aids
- ◆ Information transfer
  - ○ Read back
  - ○ Making sure that what you say is heard
- ◆ Group behaviour and complacency (smelling smoke in a group)

Environment

- ◆ Expectation bias of where you are (day-case private sector versus acute emergency-department setting)
- ◆ Situational awareness and the influence of location

Equipment

- ◆ Familiarity with equipment and when to use it, not just how to use it

Personal

- ◆ Expectation bias in a routine setting, complacency versus always expecting the unexpected
- ◆ Transitions from the routine to the emergency and back again

Personality types, learning styles, and preferred team roles

Each person undertakes a full MBTI (Myers–Briggs Type Indicator) session. We explore how this is an important tool for self-awareness. We explore the differences in preferred styles and I encourage all of those who have not yet completed an emotional intelligence (EQ) questionnaire to do so. (This

MBTI and EQ exploration is one of the parts of the course that has evolved and now forms a larger part of the training.)

I give an overview of Honey and Mumford's preferred learning styles using the camera analogy and again encourage people to undergo the formal training. I particularly encourage educators to undertake this as it makes teaching easier if you know your preferred learning style. It can explain why you find a particular student difficult to engage with, and how you may need to adjust your teaching to suit his or her needs.

I give a broad overview of Belbin's thinking[6] and again encourage people to explore this in more depth after the course has finished.

In our experience, between one-quarter and one-half of the NHS professionals who attend this level course will already be familiar with these personal development tools. We must therefore strike the balance between providing a refresher for them and new material for the others. It is worth conducting a straw poll at the beginning of this session to gauge what your starting point ought to be.

Generating new ideas (as per basic course) repeated here
Any unanswered questions?

We refer back to our original learning objectives and attempt to answer any unanswered questions.

Closure: As per basic course

I am very wary of the usual educational tool that people use at the end of courses. Like many educators I cynically call it the 'happy sheet'. We have tried to beef ours up a bit to be more thought-provoking in the hope that we encourage and capture a deeper reflection on the two-day experience.

Our 'happy sheet' also encourages participants to think about what changes they will make in their working lives and what else they might need to find out to take things forward. We use a similar Likert scale both before and after the course in an attempt to assess whether attendees are more confident in human factors knowledge, skills, and tools after the course.

After the course: As per the basic course
Summary of the course contents

Included in Table 8.2 is a breakdown of the high-level course content for both basic and advanced level matched to the SHEEP model.

Table 8.2 Human-factors course components

	Systems	Human interaction	Equipment	Environment	Personal
Basic	Culture (blame versus open) Context-specific stories Adverse event management 'Never' events Human error and hero Learn from good practice and positives Foresight/mindfulness Common language and purpose Professionalism SOPs Raising concerns	Hierarchy issues—authority gradients Team dynamics Transitions Conflict resolution Praise and respect Apology, candour Closed-loop communication Psychological safety, support Shared mental models Speaking up Non-technical skills	Standardization Compatibility IT infrastructure Human/computer interactions Proper preparation/rehearsal Right piece for patient Have you been trained in how to use this? Wide concept of equipment	Ergonomics Physical environment Interruptions Familiarity with surroundings	Self-awareness Human performance Limitations Cognitive aids Professionalism Accountability/responsibility Person-centred care Attitude Empathy Resilience
Advanced	Simplification without oversimplification Standardization Identify the 'hot spots' System analysis Measurement methodology Links with patient safety System level communication or information flow High reliability organizations Learning culture System thinking	Briefing and debriefing Leadership and 'followership' How to build a team How to change behaviour in others Provide tools Interpersonal and feedback skills Non-technical skills—more detail Double-loop learning	Procurement Design	Ergonomics—more detail	Open disclosure Developing insight Expectation bias Emotional intelligence

Source: data from 'Introduction to Human Factors', *NHS Education for Scotland*, <http://www.nes.scot.nhs.uk/education-and-training/by-theme-initiative/patient-safety-and-clinical-skills/introduction-to-patient-safety/introduction-to-human-factors.aspx>,[10] accessed 6 February 2015.

A 'train the trainer' course

I firmly believe that healthcare is different from the aviation industry (and other high-reliability organizations). Whilst I am pleased that we can learn from other industries, we do have enough brilliant trainers in healthcare with sufficient and more relevant experience. Please make use of them!

Faculty selection

Choosing faculty members who are positive role models for others is important; being a good role model is vital to their credibility in teaching human factors. This type of role model is different from being a knowledgeable trainer in a given field or perhaps being good at passing on technical skills. I recruit someone, partially at least, for their value system, and yes, I sometimes get it wrong!

Which values might I be interested in when I am recruiting?

Essential criteria

My belief is that these individuals should already be experienced educators. I want to know that they operate within a fairly level hierarchy in their primary role. I want them to be natural optimists. I want enthusiasm and an ability to generate a safe learning environment. I want them to be able to cope with tears, anger, stress, and a high cognitive workload. I want empathy and kindness. I want them to love learning and, of course, be passionate about education. I need them to believe in multi-professional training and ideally to have experience in it. I want them to be able to challenge unacceptable behaviour. I want them to demonstrate clear information transfer and great listening skills. I want them to be able to practise what we preach about team working. I want them to be from a healthcare background. And I want them to have a dollop more enthusiasm for good measure. As I believe in learning through laughter, I'd like them to be able to generate a sense of fun and have a sense of humour.

Desirable

Ideally they will be an experienced educator with pre-existing debriefing skills. Simulation experience would also be useful.

Key points on teaching human factors in healthcare

◆ Human factors course attendance is something that I think should be compulsory for all in healthcare (as it is in other high reliability organizations).

◆ The trainers should be experienced healthcare professionals with a full understanding of healthcare errors, the diversity of teams, and ways of working across our sector.

◆ The trainers should be good role models of safety positive behaviours.

◆ Trying to alter behaviour using education requires an experienced facilitator and is best achieved in small groups with face-to-face interaction. It needs to be experiential.

◆ The training should be multi-professional, with clinical and non-clinical staff training together, as well as different types of clinical professional in the training group.

◆ Enough time should be allowed for the training so that it can have the desired effect. This should never be just a box-ticking exercise and it *does not* lend itself to e-learning.

◆ There should be a basic-level course for everyone in healthcare.

◆ There should be an advanced-level course for those in leadership roles.

◆ There should be a 'train the trainer' course for those who are going to teach it. It is not a given that just anyone can nor should teach human factors skills.

◆ The situations that arise while teaching human factors can be of a delicate nature; for example, discussion of local errors and mistakes, personality interactions, bullying, or staff in difficulty. These topics require an experienced facilitator who can provide the appropriate level of support.

◆ There should be a system in place to encourage and enable sustained learning so that the course is seen as a starting point for continuous learning.

Closure

What do you know now that you didn't know when you started the book?

What are you going to do with that knowledge?

What will be your first steps?

When will you take them?

What would success look like?

How will you share it?

We have come to the end of this second book on the topic of human factors. I hope that it has been useful and enjoyable. I have recently had the wonderful news that one of the stories I related in the first book has saved its first life.

I welcome your feedback. I am happy to support as many people as I can with ideas about how to set up courses. I also run a 'train the trainer' course if the taster included is of interest.

You can get in touch with me via my website: <http://www.rlassociates.net>[9] and I can be found on LinkedIn.

I have recently set up a blog with real errors from which we can all learn and I hope to ask people to send me their errors. Let me know what you think of this idea or if you have a better one!

A final thought

I hope that you will join me in my attempts to expand human factors knowledge across the healthcare sector. I need your help to generate a passion for learning, a passion for continuous improvement, and a belief that we can all make a difference.

Thank you.

References

1. Human Factors in Healthcare. In: Board NQ, November 2013. Available at: <www.england.nhs.uk/wp-content/uploads/.../nqb-hum-fact-concord.pdf>.
2. Seaman DF, Fellenz RA. *Effective Strategies for Teaching Adults*. Columbus, OH: Merrill Publishing Co. 1989.

3. Honey P. *The Learning Styles Questionnaire: 80-item version*. Maidenhead: Peter Honey Publications, 2006.

4. Kolb DA. *Experiential Learning: Experience as the Source of Learning and Development*. Englewood Cliffs, NJ: Prentice Hall, 1984.

5. Heifetz R. *Leadership Without Easy Answers*. Cambridge, MA: Belknap Press of Harvard University Press, 1994.

6. Belbin M. *Management Teams*. London: Heinemann, 2001.

7. See the website of the Clinical Human Factors group: <http://chfg.org/>.

8. <http://www.patientstories.org.uk>.

9. <http://www.rlassociates.net>.

10. <http://www.nes.scot.nhs.uk/education-and-training/by-theme-initiative/patient-safety-and-clinical-skills/introduction-to-patient-safety/introduction-to-human-factors.aspx>.

Appendix 1

The SHEEP sheet (Figure A.1)

Systems

CULTURE

HOSPITAL CULTURE
- [ ] Departmental
- [ ] Professional
- [ ] Work group
- [ ] Mgmt vs. clinical
- [ ] Leadership culture

CULTURAL SYSTEMS
LACK OF
- [ ] Open culture
- [ ] Safety culture
- [ ] Reporting culture
- [ ] Learning culture

INFORMATION FLOW
PROBLEM WITH
- [ ] Face to face
- [ ] Phone
- [ ] Written
  - [ ] Email
  - [ ] Text
  - [ ] Notes
  - [ ] Letter/fax
- [ ] Information gathering
- [ ] Access to info systems
- [ ] Access to info sets
- [ ] Briefing
- [ ] De-briefing
- [ ] Handover
- [ ] Info transfer between
  - [ ] Individuals
  - [ ] Departments
  - [ ] Organizations

INFORMATION SYSTEMS

MANUAL
- [ ] Patient notes
- [ ] Clinical pathway
- [ ] Care bundles

AUTOMATED APLICATION
- [ ] Theatre mgmt
- [ ] Bed mgmt
- [ ] Pathology
- [ ] Patient mgmt
- [ ] Radiology

INFRASTRUCTURE
- [ ] Network
- [ ] Hardware

PRESCRIBED (SOP/Protocol/Guildline Issue)
- [ ] Failure to follow
  - [ ] National
  - [ ] Local
  - [ ] Legal & binding
  - [ ] WHO checklist
  - [ ] Care bundle
  - [ ] Research
  - [ ] Professional body
- [ ] Lack of familiarity
- [ ] Different versions
- [ ] Ambiguity within
- [ ] Ambiguity between
- [ ] Unable to locate
- [ ] Chose to deviate due to
  - [ ] Experience
  - [ ] Out of date
  - [ ] Inappropriate to situation
- [ ] Refusal to use
- [ ] Complexity
- [ ] Not understood

MODELS/TOOLS
LACK OF USE OF:
- [ ] Productive ward
- [ ] TPOT (the productive operating theatre)
- [ ] Lean/6Sigma
- [ ] SBAR
- [ ] Read back
- [ ] Active identification
- [ ] Cross check
- [ ] Risk assessment
- [ ] Time checks
- [ ] Cognitive aids
- [ ] Site/side check

ORGANIZATIONAL FLOW
PROBLEM WITH
- [ ] Clinical Department
- [ ] Business Department
- [ ] HR Department
  - [ ] Recruitment
  - [ ] Retention
- [ ] Finance Department
- [ ] IT Department
- [ ] Discharge

Human interaction

TEAM DYNAMICS & CONFLICT

PROBLEMS WITH TEAM
- [ ] Personality types
- [ ] Unclear team roles
- [ ] Preferred team role
- [ ] Perceived unfairness
- [ ] Accountability
- [ ] Approach to change
- [ ] Difference in learning/communication styles
- [ ] Lack of support
- [ ] Mixed messages/ambiguity
- [ ] Assumptions

PROBLEM STAFFING THE TEAM
- [ ] Skill mix
- [ ] Staffing level
- [ ] Staff availability

CONFLICT
- [ ] Patient interaction
- [ ] Relative interaction
- [ ] Carer interaction
- [ ] Staff interaction

PROBLEM WITH
- [ ] Leadership styles
- [ ] Lack of leadership
- [ ] Lack of followership
- [ ] Hierarchy too steep
- [ ] Hierarchy too flat

LACK OF TEAM:
- [ ] Knowledge
- [ ] Skills
- [ ] Shared mental model
- [ ] Shared decision-making

BEHAVIOURS

INTERACTION QUALITY
- [ ] Failure to challenge negative behaviour
- [ ] Lack of diversity/prejudice
- [ ] Aggression
- [ ] Laziness/apathy
- [ ] Rudeness
- [ ] Snobbery
- [ ] Dishonesty
- [ ] Lack of consideration
- [ ] Lack of respect
- [ ] Over familiarity
- [ ] Empire building
- [ ] Trying to impress
- [ ] Negativity
- [ ] Unwillingness
- [ ] Fear/insecurity
- [ ] Malicious intent

TASK

PROBLEM WITH:
- [ ] Workload/multiple
- [ ] Tasks
- [ ] Prioritization
- [ ] Allocation of tasks
  Task:
  - [ ] Incomplete
  - [ ] Quality
  - [ ] Misunderstood

SITUATIONAL AWARENESS
- [ ] Loss of sense of time
- [ ] Failure to plan ahead
- [ ] Lack of care/compassion/dignity

PROBLEMS WITH COMMUNICATION QUALITY

PROBLEM WITH:
- [ ] Delivery of message
- [ ] Lack of clarification
- [ ] Duplication/ambiguity
- [ ] Listening ability
- [ ] Body language
- [ ] Language barrier
- [ ] Understanding
- [ ] Use of pronouns
- [ ] Memory
  Lack of:
  - [ ] Commentating
  - [ ] Option generation
  - [ ] Review of decision
  - [ ] Review of diagnosis

Environment

LOCATION CHANGE

PROBLEMS WITH JOURNEY BETWEEN LOCATIONS
- [ ] Complexity
- [ ] Distance
- [ ] Accessibility
  - [ ] Size
  - [ ] Secure areas
- [ ] Modality of transfer
  - [ ] Foot
  - [ ] Chair
  - [ ] Trolley/bed/stretcher
  - [ ] Vehicle
  - [ ] Lift/elevator
  - [ ] Lifting device (hoist)

INTERRUPTIONS
- [ ] People
- [ ] Bleeps/pager
- [ ] Phones
- [ ] Machines/equipment
- [ ] Media (text, email)

PHYSICAL

PROBLEMS WITH
- [ ] Atmospheric composition (air)
- [ ] Temperature
- [ ] Humidity
- [ ] Smell
- [ ] Lighting
- [ ] Noise
- [ ] Cleanliness
- [ ] Size
- [ ] Security
- [ ] Tidiness

ERGONOMICS

PHYSICAL DESIGN PROBLEMS WITH
- [ ] Infrastructure (walls etc)
- [ ] Immovable structures (cupboards)
- [ ] Movable structures (beds, chairs)

TASK RELATED DESIGN PROBLEMS WITH
- [ ] Resource location
- [ ] Knowing where it is
- [ ] Visibility
- [ ] Accessible
- [ ] Organised
- [ ] Standardised
- [ ] Optimised

SAFETY CONTROLS
- [ ] Radiation
- [ ] Electromagnetic field (eg MRI, laser)
- [ ] Biochemical hazard

FUNCTIONAL DESIGN PROBLEMS WITH
- [ ] Proximity to eating/resting/physiological function areas
- [ ] Privacy

VICINITY
- [ ] Arms reach area
- [ ] Immediate vicinity (no doors)
- [ ] Departmental area
- [ ] Hospital/GP practice/clinical unit
- [ ] External

Figure A.1 The SHEEP 2 sheet

Equipment

GENERIC PROBLEM WITH EQUIPMENT ITSELF

- Fitness for task
- Manufacturing
- Supply
- Storage
- Availability
  - Location
  - Not in stock
  - Timely access
- Readiness for use
  - Cleanliness
  - Working order
  - Maintained
- Accuracy
- Reliability
- Safety
- Equipment compatibility
  - Electrical
- Safety coding
  - Colour
  - Device interconnection
- Model of equipment
- Equipment failure

CONSUMABLES

- Sterility
- Shelf life
- Administer
  - Wrong patient
  - Wrong consumable
  - Incompatible
  - Left in patient

DRUGS

- Prescribing abbreviated
- Prescribing illegible
- Prescribing wrong drug
- Prescribing wrong dose
- Prescribing wrong frequency
- Interactions between drugs
- Duplication
- Multiple charts
- Ambiguity
  - Dispensing
  - Preparation
  - Administer
- Wrong patient
- Wrong drug
- Wrong route
- Time delay
- Frequency
  - Too frequent
  - Too infrequent
- Wrong dose
- Wrong equipment
- Wrong technique
- Not available

NON CONSUMABLES

- Bed design
- Bed mechanical failure
- Bed electrical failure
- Bed mattress problem
- Bedrails
- Shower curtains
- Other

PROBLEM WITH USER INTERACTION WITH EQUIPMENT

- Knowledge/skill
  - Training
  - Experience
  - Frequency of use
  - Familiarity
  - Ability to troubleshoot
- Personal preference for equipment
- Availability of back-up equipment
- Ergonomic design/layout
  - User interface
  - Ease of use
  - Complexity
  - Readability
- Processing information
- Acting on information
- Post procedures check

INSTRUMENTS

- Sterility
- Administer
  - Wrong patient
  - Wrong instrument
  - Incompatible
  - Left in patient
  - Wrong site/side

MEDICAL GASES

- Prescribing
- Administer
  - Wrong patient
  - Wrong gas
  - Wrong delivery method
  - Wrong time

HUMAN TISSUE, BLOOD PRODUCTS & TRANSPLANTATION

- Collection
- Processing
- Prescribing
- Preparation
  - Cross matching
  - Other preparation
- Administer
  - Wrong patient
  - Wrong blood/ product/organ
  - Wrong route
  - Wrong time
    - Point
    - Delay
    - Duration
- Wrong dose

- Patient monitor failure

IMPLANTS/ PROSTHESES

PROBLEM WITH:
- Functionality
- Insertion method
- Wrong one
- Wrong site

2

Personal

EXTERNAL INFLUENCES

PROBLEMS WITH
- Mood
- Frustration
- Emotional security
- Emotional trigger (events)
- Feeling unprepared
- Failure to achieve expectations
- Lack of self awareness
- Confidence
- Self esteem
- Motivation
- Lack of interest
- Complacency
- Denial of the situation
- Adaptability
- Ability to cope with major change
- Distractions
- Coping with interruptions

PROBLEMS INFLUENCED BY WHO YOU ARE
- Race
- Gender
- Sexuality
- Age
- Personal value systems
- Personality (MBTI)
- Morals
- Cultural identity

PATHOLOGY/PHYSIOLOGY

- Tired
- Hungry
- Thirsty
- Toilet break
- Health/illness
  - Physical
  - Mental
- Stressed
- No energy
- Hormones/pregnancy

LIFE EVENTS

- Children
- Family
- Relationships
- Divorce
- Bereavement
- House move
- An argument
- Friends
- Commuting
- Parking
- Addiction to drugs
- Addiction to alcohol

ATTITUDES, BEHAVIOUR & EMOTION

MY WORK
PROBLEMS WITH
- An argument
- Poor morale
- Time pressure
- Lack of planning time
- Work time
- Rest time
- Work/rest balance
- Time of day
- Shift pattern
- Task conditions
  - Elective
  - Scheduled
  - Urgent
  - Emergency
  - Clinical
  - Non clinical
- High workload
- Lack of job satisfaction
- Job security
- Lack of team fit
- Lack of sense of belonging

Index